Are You Hormone Curious?

The Science of Hormone Therapy for Men and Women Explained

by

Carolyn Zaumeyer, MSN, APRN

Are You Hormone Curious?
The Science of Hormone Therapy
for Men and Women Explained

www.carolynzaumeyer.com

Author: Carolyn Zaumeyer

Cover Design: Liam Beale

Layout Design: Richard Powell

Editing, Proofreading: Carol Ferias

Publishing Service: Digital Authors LLC,
www.digital-authors.com

Table of Contents

Dedication

This book is dedicated to my husband, Alex. He has been my greatest supporter in both my personal and professional endeavors, playing a crucial role in the growth of my practice and enabling me to assist countless patients. He has accompanied me to all my speaking engagements—of which there have been many—and could deliver my presentation without notes!

As a vital member of the LowTE Florida team, we have transformed LowTE Florida into an International Center of Excellence in Bioidentical Hormone Therapy.

Thank you, Alex, for your unwavering love and support. You have made this journey extraordinary and an absolute joy!

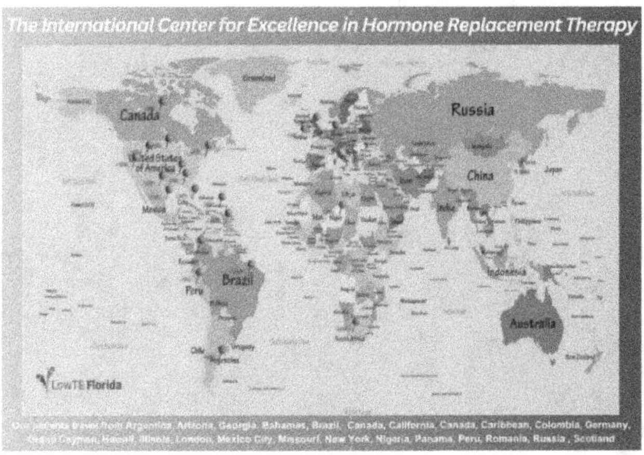

Over the years we have been amazed at how many people travel to LowTE Florida for hormone optimization.

This map represents patients that travel to LowTE Florida for treatment from around the world.

Thank you to all our patients who have traveled from near and far to LowTE Florida for their hormone optimization journey; your trust and commitment inspire us every day.

Foreword

Are you hormone curious?

When prospective patients come into the lobby at LowTE Florida in Fort Lauderdale, Florida, they see a banner with some of the possible symptoms of low hormones. The banner lists:

- Difficulty Sleeping
- Lack of Energy and Fatigue
- Reduced Mental Focus
- Moody, Anxious and Depressed
- Muscle and/or Joint Pain
- Decreased Muscle Strength
- Reduced Sexual Desire and Performance
- Weight Gain, Especially Around the Mid-Section
- Inability to Lose Weight, Regardless of Diet and Exercise

Several patients have said: "Can I have a marker so I can mark off ***all the symptoms*** listed on the banner?" Everyone's experience with declining hormones is different. That is the beauty of what I do I personalize the dosing of our treatment tailored specifically for you.

- So, let's get started answering the questions I hear every day from prospective patients.

- What are hormones?

- What do they do?

- Is hormone therapy something I should consider?

- What are the health benefits of aging with hormones?

- Is HRT safe?

- Why aren't my doctors recommending hormone therapy for me?

I hope to answer your questions and help you feel more comfortable as you begin to get back to your "old self" safely and comfortably.

Carolyn Zaumeyer

STORIES OF TRANSFORMATION

"**A Personal Tribute**" by MEV/RV (husband and wife)

Dear Readers,

What an honor and privilege it is for me—or I guess us (me and hubby)—to write some words for this amazing rock star of a woman, Carolyn Zaumeyer, who has probably helped hundreds of women, men, and couples live their best life with her quest to provide the best hormone replacement therapy available. Her vast knowledge and continued passion to help us feel our best as we reach our next phase in life is admirable and exciting. I hope this book continues to help answer any questions and dispel the misconceptions that are out there confusing people about hormone replacement therapy.

So, here we are, mid-50s, married almost 30 years! Yes, daunting and sometimes I'm like "What the heck? And how are we so happy?" Love of course, is the best answer, but how about the rest of how marriage should be after 25 or 30 years? I was lucky enough to meet a friend back in 2017, who after 5 minutes of chatting about life and being a full-time working mother, wife and trying to meet so many expectations for myself and others as a super woman, I was so very tired by 3:00 p.m. and not ready for the second half of what the day had waiting for me.

This is when my life changed. This friend referred me to Carolyn for a consultation about hormone replacement therapy. Now, today, in 2024, I have never looked back! After about my second therapy appointment, I was a different woman. My energy level, my sleep, my interest in sex and fitness were once again a huge part of my life. My menopausal mood swings—sometimes rage—were in the past. I was me again.

My husband was so taken aback at my change, he was definitely curious and did not want to be left behind (smart man). He was lacking the energy for physical fitness and definitely the libido was not how he wanted it to be. So, I went with him to have a little chat with Carolyn, and that was that. HE also has never looked back! HE is back to the guy I married—actually even better. ☺

Our lives changed. We became happy and balanced empty-nesters, excited for life, travel, adventure, and our love and attraction has grown. The stress of life is there of course, but handled completely different. We feel our lives have been restored somehow to when it all began—a second chance at enjoying each other's company and looking forward to our lives together.

We are so thankful to Carolyn for helping us through our journey entering our second phase of life—we love her energy and her positivity at every appointment. Love hearing her always tell us "Continue to have rockin' sex…"

"Our Journey to Hormone Balance" by Emily and Tom

Emily and I (Tom) began to be aware of our lack of hormone balance when we were in our upper 40s. After Emily's hysterectomy (she kept her ovaries), she experienced a dry and thinning vagina, discomfort during sex, and a complete lack of libido. I had a bout of hyperthyroidism, a lack of energy, as well as moderate insomnia, and my ability to think became sluggish.

Fortunately, Emily's OB/GYN at the time was a bit of a free thinker, and started her on HRT, albeit with synthetic hormones (Premarin). The estrogen helped a little with the vaginal symptoms but did nothing for her libido. When he suggested that her lack of libido might be helped by testosterone, we were shocked! Testosterone for a woman? He encouraged us to give it a try and he gave her a testosterone injection.

Wow! Her libido was intense for about a week, and then pfft! It was gone again! We learned that the testosterone shots don't work for very long. Meanwhile, I had my testosterone tested and it was 166 when optimally it should be in the 800 range.

So, we had identified the problem in both of us: low testosterone. But what was the solution? Emily tried Estratest®, another synthetic hormone, and that helped, but it didn't produce the results we knew were possible, plus we were learning about the potential dangers of synthetic hormones and wanted a healthier solution. I tried a testosterone cream from a compounding pharmacy. That somewhat improved my testosterone, pushing it up into the 300-400 range, but I had to rub the greasy stuff into my quadriceps once a day, and that skin couldn't touch anyone else (like my grandchildren) or it might OD them! Marginal results, and very inconvenient.

I'm a distance runner, and I also fly a lot for work, so when an athletic-looking gentleman about my age with high-tech running shoes sat down next to me on a flight, I naturally asked him if he was a runner, which started a conversation that changed our lives! He told me that he and his wife had started bioidentical hormone replacement therapy pellets, and since then, not only was he having a lot more fun running, but he and his wife's intimate relationship had skyrocketed, which he illustrated by sharing that they had had sex four times in the previous two days! Obviously, I pumped him for all the information he could give me! When I got home to Illinois, I searched and searched and found out that no one anywhere near us had any idea what I was talking about. I then wondered if it was real or not.

A few weeks later, Emily and I were in Fort Lauderdale, Florida, and I was preparing to run the A1A Half Marathon in January of 2017. As usual, we attended the pre-race Expo, visiting the various vendors, when we came upon a booth for "LowTE Florida." Instantly intrigued, I began to pepper the two helpful women with my questions! I soon realized; this was exactly the bioidentical pellet therapy that the fellow on the flight had told me about! They offered us a free consultation, which we eagerly accepted.

Carolyn patiently listened to our story and began to teach us about optimizing our hormones using bioidentical pellets inserted in our hips a couple of times a year. She explained that this type of therapy had been in successful use since the 1930s! This vital information, which she has now painstakingly compiled in this book, fit hand-in-glove with everything we had been learning over the previous 20 years; it completed the puzzle! At that moment we wondered if it was too good to be true. Could this method of hormone replacement therapy give us the results we had been searching for over a decade? And would it accomplish its goals day after day, week after week, with no spikes or lulls, and no daily fuss nor muss? Now, more than 7 years later, we are in our upper 60s and the answer is an unqualified: YES!

I have an extremely mentally challenging professional career, and for the past 7+ years of pellet therapy by Carolyn, my thinking processes have remained sharp. As a matter of fact, the way I know when my pellets need to be renewed is when my mentation starts to slow down! Emily's vagina is healthy and self-lubricating, and her libido is now stronger than it's ever been in our 49 years of marriage. Our sexual relationship is more active than it's ever been, we enjoy sex 4 or 5 times a week, and for both of us, our orgasms are more intense than ever before in our lives. It's wonderful! Plus, now I fall asleep within a minute of laying my head on the pillow... every night!

On a final note, 2 or 3 times a year we travel from our home in Illinois to Fort Lauderdale, Florida (where Carolyn and LowTE Florida are located) to get our pellets inserted. But it's totally worth it because, as you will discover in this book, Carolyn is the "Maestro of pellets!" I encourage you to read this volume from cover to cover and see just how much the quality of your daily life can be improved! It certainly has for us!

Foreword

"A Professional Endorsement" by Douglas Caporrino

Dear Future Patient,

My name is Doug Caporrino, I'm a functional medicine nutritionist author and bio chemist. I can tell you in my 40 years plus in the wellness industry I rarely come across practitioners that I recommend. I can tell you without a doubt that Carolyn Zaumeyer is one of my goto practitioners. I've been sending patients to her for years. I can tell you without hesitation, that her integrity, intellect, and overall compassion is second to none. I always say the proof is in the results, and Carolyn gets results, plain and simple.

I have always believed that HRT is necessary in one's life, depending on the time and circumstances. If I were to trust anyone with my HRT, or that of a loved one, I would highly recommend Carolyn.

Yours in health,

Douglas Caporrino, CNS, MBS

Prologue
My Journey

Before we get into the heart of this book (the many aspects of anti-aging healthcare that I deliver faithfully to my patients at my LowTE Florida practice in Fort Lauderdale, Florida), I suppose good manners dictate that I introduce myself a bit and tell you what brought me to this field in the first place.

I have been asked many times: "Why have you devoted your life and career to bioidentical hormones?"

A good and fair question! After all, if your healthcare provider isn't truly passionate about doing everything in their power to help you achieve your health and wellness goals, it's time to look for a new professional to manage your care.

Let me assure you I am passionate about optimizing my patients' health. And, as you'll see in short order, the proof is in the pudding in the results that I deliver day-in, day-out in my hands-on clinical practice.

I could be working in many less controversial areas of medicine than the anti-aging field, however, since my professional passion is getting people to feel their best as they age, here I am.

It's no secret, as we'll explore in this book, that modern institutionalized medicine, while excellent in many areas, is lacking. In many cases, simple and affordable interventions like bioidentical hormone replacement therapy, thyroid optimization, and targeted nutritional supplementation (of course, along with some lifestyle changes) are the missing links to optimal health that patients who come to my LowTE Florida office aren't even aware of—because their general practice doctor never enlightened them! I fill in the gaps, providing my patients with the anti-aging tools and education they need to truly thrive.

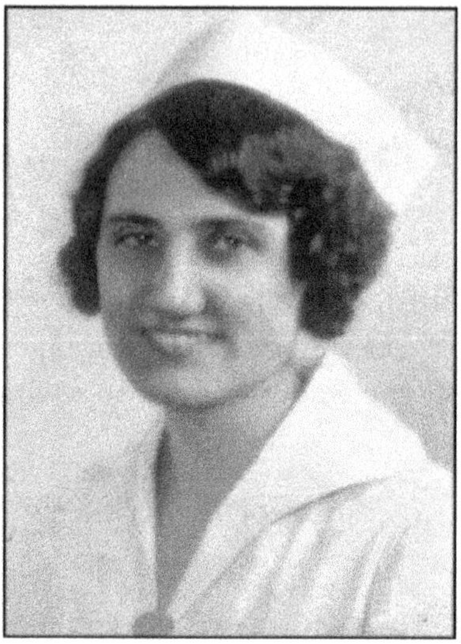

This dedication to patient care stems from my early inspiration to become a nurse. My passion for nursing was sparked at a young age, thanks to my Great Aunt Edna. She graduated nursing school in the 1920s in Chicago and, in a bold adventure, drove to California in a Model T Ford to become a "Nurse to the Stars!" I fondly remember her visiting our farm and sharing fabulous stories about her experiences, including caring for celebrities like Clark Gable. Her enthusiasm inspired me to pursue nursing, and I've never regretted that decision.

This foundation in nursing led me to explore various specialties, eventually guiding me to anti-aging medicine. So, how did I come to this field?

My path to anti-aging healthcare has been serendipitous. When I first graduated from the Nurse Practitioner program at Florida International University in 1992, I was very fortunate to have been hired by a physician who specialized in Obstetrics and Gynecology.

I was like a little sponge, soaking up as much of his knowledge and treatment plans as I could.

I was in Heaven! Until… when completing chart reviews, I noticed a trend with the menopausal patients: oftentimes, in the physician's notes, would often be written the ominous phrase "psych referral."

I was perplexed; how could all these women need to see a psychiatrist? It's not that I don't believe the field of psychiatry is legitimate or that we shouldn't seek counseling when it's needed, but how could a psych referral be the first-resort treatment for women who were clearly struggling with the very real physical and emotional effects of menopause, mediated by hormonal disruptions? It didn't add up.

So, I stacked up the charts and carried them to the physician, my boss, and asked why he was referring them to a psychiatrist. "They are miserable, crying, they are sweaty, and their relationships are a mess! They need to get their lives together!" was his reply.

I asked, "Can I please have these patients?"

"God bless you! You can have them. You take care of the old birds, and I will deliver babies," he said.

PERFECT, I thought. That is when it all started to come together for me. I started correcting menopausal women's varied health issues, both mental and physical, with the traditional medications available, and I got incredible feedback.

I recall one patient who called me and said she wanted to thank me for giving her, her life back! She liked herself more, her husband liked her more, and life was just more fun! And then came another similar phone call, and then another. That experience was the match that lit the fire of my passion for hormone optimization, and I've been off to the races ever since.

I was happily treating my menopausal patients with traditional hormone replacement therapy until 2002, when the devastating report of the findings from a study by the Women's Health Initiative came out—a dubious study that we'll break down later in this book. A single study, built on a flawed design and later heavily critiqued for its misleading conclusions, blew my synthetic hormones out of the water!

Virtually overnight, 80% of American women went off their hormones due to the fear induced by media reporting that hormone replacement caused breast cancer. This was a very troubling assertion, one that I had to get to the bottom of. After much subsequent research, talented clinical researchers have demonstrated that the ***synthetic progestin*** used in the original study that had been paired with Premarin, (rather than therapeutic progesterone) was the culprit causing all the problems reported.

So, given the potential risks of combining synthetic hormones in therapy, how was I going to care for all my patients who were thriving on hormone therapy?

I found the answer in bioidentical hormone replacement therapy (BHRT)—as opposed to the conventional, synthetic Big Pharma drugs I had been prescribing previously.

And, yes, there is a world of difference between synthetic and bioidentical hormones. Like comparing apples and oranges. We're going to dig deep here to prove it.

The transition from synthetic to bioidentical hormones in therapy was a big step for me. Bioidentical hormones were, much to the detriment of patients, not discussed at all in nursing school or medical school curricula at that time. (To this day, in fact, the hormones are woefully neglected healthcare provider training.)

I decided that, if I was going to go in this new direction, I needed to develop the confidence that I was prescribing the right hormones with the right dosing and the safest delivery systems.

In that pursuit, I sought out the nation's most knowledgeable experts on bioidentical hormones. I traveled throughout the country to study with them. With each visit, I would always return home ready and excited to apply my new knowledge.

Still, through all my hands-on research with the profession's best hormone care providers, the optimal dosing instruction had still not been crystallized until I studied under Dr. Gary Donovitz. He is a brilliant teacher who was able to fill in my gaps of knowledge and gave me the confidence that I could provide hormone replacement safely. I credit him with teaching me how to dose hormones precisely and I will be forever grateful to him for sharing his vast knowledge over the years.

With all this extensive research and clinical background under my belt, I launched LowTE Florida in 2013 in Fort Lauderdale, Florida. My practice has enjoyed astronomical growth, so much so that I was just included in the Healthcare Business Review Top Ten Hormone Therapy Providers in the nation for the past two years.

Writing a book to educate and entertain both patients and other providers is, admittedly, a formidable task. My goal with this work is to dispel the many myths and misconceptions about bioidentical hormone therapy that to this day continue to confuse many people, largely due to lack of knowledge by current healthcare providers, a lack of proper training for up-and-coming providers, and inaccurate media reporting.

As I mentioned earlier, the proof of my expertise in this area of medicine, as the saying goes, "is in the pudding." I see new patients every day who are not feeling well. After treatment, to quote many patients, they "feel like [their] old selves!", "have a better sense of well-being" and many times "this is life changing!".

I love my work. I see people who are not feeling well, I give them hope, and then, together, using the clinical knowledge I have built over many years and standing on the shoulders of giants like Dr. Donovitz, Dr. Neil Rouzier, Dr. Daved Rosensweet, Dr. Lindsey Berkson, Dr. Angela DeRosa and Dr. Terri DeNeui. We are able to restore their good health, turning back the clock 10-15 years.

Love it!

Chapter I

Slaying the Chronic Disease Dragon

When the medical history of this period is written, the verdict will be clear: Overall, we have failed as a profession in the developed world to provide the kind of *wellness* care (not sick care) that our patients need to not just survive but to *thrive*.

My mission as an Advanced Registered Nurse Practitioner on the medical frontlines is to help set things right in that respect. My career is devoted to helping real patients like you achieve optimal health daily in my clinical practice.

Right from the start, let's be careful to not throw the baby out with the bathwater: there are many things that modern Western medicine does *right*—and not just right, but *excellently*.

Nothing is black and white; we should be proud of our achievements as medical professionals while recognizing areas where we can do better. After all, we can walk and chew gum at the same time, as they say!

For instance, if you have a broken limb or some other traumatic injury from, for example, a car accident (a common occurrence in our fast-paced world), there are few places you would rather be than in a top-notch American medical facility, entrusted to the skilled hands of well-trained trauma care providers.

Likewise, modern medicine has done a commendable job at limiting, mitigating, and in some cases fully eradicating infectious illness, such as polio and smallpox, among many others.

With that caveat aside, there is much that modern medicine gets *wrong*—first and foremost, the prevention, treatment, and reversal of chronic illnesses, a broad category that includes heart disease, autoimmune disease, cancer, and neurodegenerative disease.

Let's start with the basics here.

The term "disease" is a contraction of the Latin prefix "dis," which, per the Merriam-Webster dictionary, means the "opposite or absence of," and "ease," which means "freedom from pain, worry, or trouble; comfort" according to Collins Dictionary.

So, "disease" is a negative condition meaning the lack of comfort or well-being.

What **disease** is *not* is a positive state; rather, it **is the absence of wellness**. The appropriate objective in treating disease, then, is to restore the state of wellness—not merely to treat whatever health condition can be diagnosed.

This is, in my view and in the view of elite anti-aging healthcare providers at the top of their game, the appropriate lens through which wellness providers like me view our practice: we use the many and growing arsenal of tools at our disposal to optimize every aspect of our patients' health in order to slow, stop, and, increasingly, in many cases, reverse the health deficits commonly accompanying the aging process.

It's not enough anymore—and we shouldn't accept it as standard care—to merely treat disease and send patients on their way. Our goal needs to be fostering a condition of overall, total wellness. We need to set our sights higher together, as providers and as patients.

The stakes couldn't be higher; the toll that chronic disease takes on Americans' quality of life is immense, as I witness the impacts firsthand in my clinical practice daily.

The clinical literature on this subject bears out what I see firsthand in many of my patients in terms of the often-devastating burden of chronic illness.

From the International Journal of Environmental Research and Public Health [1]:

> ***"Nearly half (approximately 45%, or 133 million) of all Americans suffer from at least one chronic disease****, and the number is growing. Chronic diseases—including, cancer, diabetes,*

hypertension, stroke, heart disease, respiratory diseases, arthritis, obesity, and oral diseases—can lead to hospitalization, long-term disability, reduced quality of life, and death. In fact, ***persistent conditions are the nation's leading cause of death and disability****."*

The numbers, tragically, don't lie; the overwhelming statistical likelihood that you or one of your family members suffers from one or more chronic illnesses is virtually guaranteed. It's just as likely that, without intervention, over time, these conditions will prove fatal.

The everyday symptoms of chronic illness are often broad-based, non-specific, and therefore clinically difficult to attribute to any one diagnosis. They include:

- Low energy
- Poor sleep (insomnia)
- Unwanted weight gain
- Fat accumulation around the hip and thighs or the gut.
- Depression
- Anxiety
- Mood swings
- Inability to focus
- Poor sexual performance (including erectile dysfunction in men and vaginal dryness in women experiencing menopause)
- Loss of interest in sex
- Loss of interest in other activities you once loved

Of course, all these symptoms have multiple possible triggers.

It is this lack of specificity in correlating symptoms to their causes, among other reasons, that the roots of chronic illness—such as **hormone imbalances**, one of the most neglected aspects of clinical medicine in many instances—all too often go unaddressed, leaving patients and their loved ones to suffer needlessly.

In the American culture, we're conditioned through advertising and other means to demand immediate results, and healthcare is no exception. In pharmaceutical advertising on television, for instance, the overriding message is: "take this pill for instant relief and all of your problems will disappear."

While this kind of messaging might help sell products, it's unfortunately extremely misleading. Treating and reversing chronic illness and, ultimately, achieving total wellness take time and effort—along with the expert guidance of an experienced provider throughout the journey.

To summarize in simpler terms, we have a crisis of chronic illness that requires a serious reorientation of how we approach healthcare. The alternative, which is unacceptable, is the continued rise in rates of chronic disease and its devastating impacts on patients' quality of life and that of their families.

If all that sounds bleak, here's the truly great news: **chronic illness is not your destiny, and it doesn't need to be your reality—not now or ever**.

There *is* a proven path back to optimal health, based on my decades of experience helping patients, and I'm going to lay out the roadmap for you here.

There are many well-vetted methods, backed by reams of clinical research, to treat and reverse chronic illness, restore optimal health, and live your best life possible even deep into your golden years.

One such method, for example, which we'll get into in much greater detail in later chapters, is hormone replacement therapy (HRT), the benefits of which are briefly elaborated upon by the medical journal Climacteric [3] for postmenopausal women:

> *"Nowadays, postmenopausal women are largely under-treated. Analysis... suggests that hormone replacement therapy (HRT) can prevent osteoporosis and cardiovascular disease in symptomatic, early postmenopausal women. In fact, climacteric [menopause] symptoms are related to an increased risk of chronic conditions, including hypertension and cardiovascular disease... HRT may prevent chronic conditions when started in symptomatic women*

before the age of 60 years or within 10 years of the onset of the menopause."

My patients range in age from 30 to 92! You are not too old to begin Bioidentical Hormone Replacement Therapy. Don't fret, men. Hormone therapy is for almost everyone! There are numerous anti-aging benefits you can reap from testosterone replacement therapy—also known by its acronym, TRT—that we'll discuss coming up as well.)

Getting to, and staying at your mental, physical, and emotional peak, even as you move through the years, is going to be the focus of this book.

My mission, again—a goal that I've helped thousands of patients achieve over the years—is to treat the underlying causes of your chronic disease and put you on a fast track to the inverse of chronic illness: not just a lack of disease, but total, chronic wellness.

If looking and feeling your absolute best—possibly decades younger than your chronological age—is what you most hope to achieve from your interactions with healthcare providers, I dedicate this book to you.

May you find healing in these pages.

Because everything I do in my clinical practice is based on rigorous scientific evidence, I will include the annotations for each source cited in this chapter and throughout this book in the "References" sections located at the end of each chapter.

References

[1] Raghupathi, W. and Raghupathi, V. (2018, March 1). An empirical study of chronic diseases in the United States: A visual analytics approach. International journal of environmental research and public health. https://www.ncbi.nlm.nih.gov/pmc/articles/PMC5876976/

[2] Reynolds, R., Dennis, S., Hasan, I., Slewa, J., Chen, W., Tian, D., Bobba, S., Zwar, N. (2018, January 9). A systematic review of chronic disease management interventions in primary care. BMC family practice. https://www.ncbi.nlm.nih.gov/pmc/articles/PMC5759778/

[3] S;, G. M. A. (n.d.). *Hormone replacement therapy and prevention of chronic conditions.* Climacteric : the journal of the International Menopause Society. https://pubmed.ncbi.nlm.nih.gov/30626218/

Chapter II

Modern Healthcare vs. Sick Care: What's the Difference and Why Does It Matter

Let me begin with a question for you, my reader and future patient: when was the last time your doctor asked, "How do you feel?" instead of "What's wrong" or "Tell me about your symptoms"?

With this single question, we encapsulate the central problem with the practice of modern medicine that I alluded to in the previous chapter: if your doctor isn't going deep into the metaphorical weeds in terms of your health status, but is instead treating symptoms on a piecemeal basis, then it's sick care, not *true* healthcare, or wellness care, as many of us in the field call it.

But what do those terms mean exactly—sick care and wellness care—and what are the differences between them that matter?

Sick care means:

- No hormone care
- No nutrition care
- No integration of healing care for the mind *and* the body
- Treating (or, often, *attempting to, but failing* to treat) the symptoms of disease instead of getting at the underlying cause
- An emphasis on (often expensive) synthetic pharmaceutical drugs as a first-resort option over more fundamental, sustainable interventions

Wellness care means:

- Hormone optimization

- Thyroid optimization
- Nutrition optimization (healthy, whole foods-based eating plans with the proper macronutrient ratios and micronutrient concentrations)
- Strategic nutritional supplementation when necessary
- An integrative approach to medicine in which we incorporate care for both the mind (and/or the spirit, if you are spiritual) and the body, as the two are inextricably linked
- A holistic, long-term healing approach with plenty of follow-up care—no shortcuts, no single-symptom treatments

The above is only a summary of the distinctions between sick care and wellness care, but as we move through this book, the differences between the competing philosophies will become increasingly clear.

To put it in layman's terms, we've come up short in our commonly accepted definition of what constitutes "health." The popular denotation of the term simply means "no disease present," whereas what we need to be striving for is much, much more: total wellness, in every aspect of life, with no compromises accepted.

We're not going to tolerate any more of the "this just comes with the aging process" excuse to explain away not feeling at your absolute peak.

There has, arguably, never been a greater need for a total paradigm shift within the medical profession from sick care to wellness care.

So, from a practical perspective, here's the difference in terms of the in-the-exam-room patient experience between sick care and wellness care.

During a sick care visit:

- Your doctor asks, "what's wrong?" or "why are you here today?"
- You tell the doctor your symptoms (fatigue, low libido, mood swings, weight gain, etc.)
- Your doctor offers a reductive intervention meant to treat single symptoms one at a time (antidepressants to treat depression or hot flashes, Viagra or Cialis to treat erectile dysfunction, etc.)

while neglecting to address deeper issues for long-term, lasting improvements in your health

During a wellness care visit at my LowTE Florida office:

- We discuss all your symptoms—including how they affect your everyday life and how you envision thriving instead of suffering—and examine how they might be interconnected
- We conduct *comprehensive* (not piecemeal) lab testing as necessary to get a true, holistic sense of what's going on in your physiology
- We leave no stone unturned to get to the heart of the matter (no pun intended)
- We develop and implement a *comprehensive* (not piecemeal) treatment plan based on your wellness goals with plenty of follow-up visits and phone calls as necessary to review progress and fine-tune our protocols for optimal results

My patients see the world of difference between sick care and wellness care when they come to me. They often can't believe how lacking their prior care was in its scope and scale—and they'll tell me they frequently didn't even know the kind of holistic, potentially life-changing wellness care that we practice at LowTE Florida was out there waiting to be discovered.

Many times, after I diagnose unknown diabetes, hypothyroidism or Hashimoto's thyroiditis I am asked, "Why didn't my primary care provider test me for this?" I tell them that is a very good question to take to their healthcare (or sick care) provider.

Not to worry! Help is on its way!

References

[1] Defining whole health - achieving whole health - NCBI bookshelf. (n.d.). https://www.ncbi.nlm.nih.gov/books/NBK591719/

[2] Fani Marvasti, F. and Stafford, R. S. (2012). From sick care to health care--reengineering prevention into the U.S. system. The New England journal of medicine. https://www.ncbi.nlm.nih.gov/pmc/articles/PMC4339086/

Chapter III

What Are Hormones and Why Do they Matter for Your Health?

The centrality of the endocrine system (aka the hormone system) to optimal human health is nearly impossible to understate.

There are more than 50 hormones present in the human body that work in harmony to perform all manner of critical activities ranging from regulating metabolism (energy processing and usage) to igniting sex drive to enhancing cognitive function.

The essential role of the hormones in human health, why paying sufficient attention to them for both patient and healthcare provider is a must, and the complex interactions between the hormones are succinctly summarized here by noted medical text StatPearls[1]:

> *"**Hormones of the endocrine system are a vast topic** with numerous hormones involved, **affecting virtually every organ in the human body.** Human **physiologic processes such as homeostasis, metabolic demand, development, and reproduction** are all possible because of hormones and the processes mediated by their actions... **Understanding how hormones interact to maintain the body tightly within the strict limits of homeostasis is imperative...Hormones are often intricately related and may influence other hormones,** which are the primary presenting symptoms."*

In a nutshell, here's how hormones work:

- Glands located in various parts of the body produce them. Such glands that comprise the human endocrine system include testes

(in men), ovaries (in women), thyroid, parathyroid, pituitary, pineal, pancreas, adrenals, and thymus.
- The glands, at regular intervals, secrete (inject) their respective hormones directly into the bloodstream, at which time they traverse the body.
- The hormones come upon their corresponding hormone receptor sites located on certain cells and bind to them.
- When they bind to the receptor sites on the cells, they then trigger desirable and necessary changes in the function of the target cells—and, at the next level of analysis, the tissues and organs that groups of cells comprise.
- Homeostasis (healthy and stable condition of the body) is maintained in this way.

Hormones are, in short, involved in nearly every physiological function known to medical science—and intimately so.

Given that there are more than 50 hormones in the body, listing them all comprehensively here would be too unwieldy a task to manage. But here are a few of what are considered the "most important" hormones in the body (although all 50+ are important) that you might have heard of:

- Estrogen (the main female sex hormone)
- Testosterone (the main male sex hormone)
- Insulin (for regulating blood sugar levels; if you or someone you love has diabetes, you're probably well-acquainted with this one)
- Cortisol (aka the "stress hormone")
- Triiodothyronine (T3) and thyroxine (T4), often simply called the thyroid hormones
- Melatonin (in charge of regulating the circadian rhythm, or the sleep/wake cycle)

So, for an illustrative rundown of the process of hormonal regulation of homeostasis from start to finish, let's briefly look at a very simple summation of the action of insulin—keeping in mind that, per the literature we've quoted above, the interaction between the totality of the hormones and the organs and tissues they work on is a highly complex interplay (after all, that's why endocrinology is a highly specialized field of medicine!).

Here's how the insulin hormone works:

- You eat a carbohydrate-containing meal or snack (for example, a piece of fruit)
- The food travels to your small intestines, where it is broken down by the digestive system
- The glucose, protein, and fat from the broken-down food enters the bloodstream
- Blood sugar rises as a result
- In response to elevated blood sugar levels, the pancreas (located next to the liver) releases insulin
- Insulin travels throughout the body, binding to cells in muscle tissue, fat tissue, and the liver
- The muscles then absorb the blood sugar and store it for later use as glycogen, the insulin signals to the liver to convert blood sugar into fatty acids, and the insulin triggers fat tissue to process and store the blood sugar as triglycerides
- In this way, insulin removes excess sugar from the blood—where you don't want it to be in the long-term—and shuttles it into the tissues and organs where it can serve a useful purpose (namely, providing immediate and stored energy)

If something goes wrong with this critical process of insulin release and regulation of blood sugar, the human organism develops what is called metabolic dysfunction—often in the form of diabetes, one of the most common chronic illnesses in the modern world.

And insulin is just one example. Indeed, the dysfunction or deficit of *any* of the hormones will lead to extremely negative health outcomes over time.

The problem with hormonal dysfunction, I hope I've done a good job of making clear by now, is well-defined and indisputable.

Now let's talk about solutions.

First, which should be obvious, you need to seek out and sync up with an expert in hormone care who knows how to properly investigate, diagnose, and effectively treat hormone imbalances.

We've established, in addition to the unfortunate lack of hormone care in sick care, that an ideal wellness protocol emphasizes hormone *optimization*, not mere clinical sufficiency, as a central objective to help patients feel and look their best.

So, let's get right into the many, proven, often life-changing benefits (many of my patients have described their health transformations not just as benefits but as "miracles") of using hormones to age with grace and vitality.

We'll begin with the general benefits (overall quality of life) and then get more specific—all the while, relying only on clinical literature from reputable sources, the details of which, again, are provided in the "References" section so you can access them at your leisure if you are interested in the original material.

Overall Quality of Life

As we'll explore here, "quality of life" [QoL] is a broad and important measurement of how well an individual is able to go about their daily routines, doing what they love and "sucking the marrow out of life," as it were.

So, to get a little terminological housekeeping out of the way, the official definition of "quality of life," as offered by StatPearls[2], is as follows:

> *"Quality of life (QoL) is a concept which aims to capture the well-being, whether of a population or individual, regarding both positive and negative elements within the entirety of their existence at a specific point in time. For example,* ***common facets of QoL include personal health (physical, mental, and spiritual), relationships, education status, work environment, social status, wealth, a sense of security and safety, freedom, autonomy in***

decision-making, social-belonging and their physical surroundings. *"*

Now, admittedly, that's a lot to pack into a single concept, but comprehensiveness is the point; there's a lot that goes into "quality of life" as a metric, and rightfully so. Life is varied and complex, after all—but you don't need a healthcare provider to tell you that!

Given the expansive definition of QoL, let's consider the results of a 2008 British Medical Journal[3] in which 3,721 women aged 50-69 were split into the experimental group (receiving HRT) and a placebo group and then surveyed on various QoL outcomes.

Here is a summary of the outcomes:

> *"In this randomized controlled trial* ***women who started taking combined HRT many years after menopause experienced improved sleep and reduced vasomotor symptoms. They also reported fewer aching joints and muscles, less vaginal dryness, and improved sexual functioning,*** *but breast tenderness and vaginal discharge increased. The beneficial changes in sleep and sexual functioning were independent of the presence of baseline vasomotor symptoms (flushes or night sweats)…*
>
> ***The results of WISDOM are clinically relevant for doctors treating postmenopausal women*** *with relevant symptoms including vasomotor symptoms, sleep disturbance, and aching joints and muscles."*

"The domains in which the replacement therapy proved significantly better were vasomotor symptoms, sexual functioning, sleep problems, night sweats, vaginal dryness, and aching joints or muscles," concurred another clinical researcher, in an article also published in 2008, in this case in Reviews in Obstetrics and Gynecology [4], remarking on the same body of research cited above.

Systematic, clinical reviews of the positive impact of HRT on QoL are legion.

But now let's get our fine-tooth comb out and explore the benefits of HRT on very particular areas of health, such as physical performance, sexual performance and satisfaction, cognitive function, etc.

Physical Performance

Whether your primary interest in pursuing HRT is in staying active in your work for as long as possible, maximizing your athletic prowess even in your golden years, or simply staying fit to play with your grandchildren—or all three! —I know firsthand, based on years of clinical experience, that physical performance is a paramount concern of aging patients.

So, let's get into what HRT does, based on the clinical literature, for physical performance.

Testosterone, the "male sex hormone", has long been understood by medical science to be critical for achieving peak physical/athletic performance for both men and women, hence the reason that many athletes supplement with testosterone, sometimes legally, but sometimes illegally using anabolic steroids. (In a later section, we'll explore the differences between bioidentical hormones and anabolic steroids and why they matter.) In fact, most sporting bodies heavily restrict or outright ban testosterone supplementation in athletes for the very reason that it can lend what many consider an unfair athletic edge over the competition.

That said, testosterone replacement therapy (TRT) for optimized physical performance isn't just for athletes, as explained via Sports Health [5]:

> *"While the performance-enhancing effects of testosterone have been known in athletic populations since the 1950s,* ***there has recently been a considerable amount of work investigating its role in aging populations****. The justification behind this work is logical:* ***Many of the more apparent changes of aging, such as loss of muscle and bone mass, libido, and energy, are often the inverse of what is reported in testosterone users****. Furthermore, it is well understood that testosterone levels decrease with normal aging.*

Thus, it follows that ***replacing testosterone in an older population may lead to reversal of some of these negative effects****...*

There is extensive research available on the effects of testosterone in the aging man and several major reviews of these studies. These data suggest that ***testosterone replacement designed to restore levels similar to the normal young man results in increased lean body mass, muscle strength, bone density, and decreased body fat, without much in the way of side effects****."*

HRT also helps women with athletic performance.

One noted study on the benefits of HRT for physical performance in women experiencing menopause was published in the medical journal Clinical Science (London)[6]. Its findings led the researchers to conclude that "in post-menopausal women, **muscle performance, muscle mass and muscle composition are improved by HRT**. The beneficial effects of HRT combined with high-impact physical training may exceed those of HRT alone."

The group that experienced the best results was the one receiving both hormone therapy *and* exercise.

Muscle Mass

Related to physical performance, a distinct benefit of HRT, particularly for older patients, is the boost in lean muscle mass that it provides.

Why should you shoot for higher muscle mass as you age? The answer is that, unfortunately, loss of muscle mass is a common feature of hormone deficiency, especially later in life—and the ramifications of not addressing it are dire.

In anti-aging medicine, we use the term "sarcopenia" to refer to age-related declines in muscle mass, as explained via clinical literature published in the medical journal Current Opinion in Rheumatology [7]:

> *"An age related, involuntary loss of skeletal muscle mass and strength.* ***Beginning as early as the 4th decade of life,*** *evidence suggests that* ***skeletal muscle mass and skeletal muscle strength decline*** *in a linear fashion, with* ***up to 50% of mass being lost by the 8th decade of life."***

Now, you don't need to be a doctor to see that a 50% decline in precious muscle mass and an accompanying loss of strength is, to put it mildly, not ideal.

Research has identified a strong causal relationship between low testosterone in men (sometimes called "androgen deficiency") and sarcopenia, as elaborated upon in this published study from The World Journal of Men's Health [8]:

> *"Aging affects metabolism, leading to physiological and functional impairments, and is also related to changes in body composition, including reduced skeletal muscle mass and increased body fat. These changes are correlated with the pathophysiology of sarcopenia, which is defined as age-related loss of skeletal muscle mass and strength.* ***Low testosterone levels are associated with unfavorable body composition changes, and sex hormones decrease with aging. Androgen deficiency****, along with lack of exercise and poor nutrition,* ***may be among the modifiable contributors to sarcopenia****."*

But the potential health consequences of sarcopenia are even worse than you might imagine at first glance, as they extend well beyond the mere loss of athletic ability and physical function. In fact, sarcopenia contributes to serious chronic illness that significantly threatens QoL and lifespan.

"Loss of muscle mass and function is correlated with high morbidity and mortality owing to an increased risk of frailty and falling... The perceived importance of muscle mass and function and overall interest in the topic have been increasing," adds The World Journal of Men's Health.

So, if you aim to not just optimize physical performance but keep metabolic dysfunction, arthritis, and other forms of chronic disease at bay, it's critical to preserve and regain lost lean muscle mass.

HRT is clinically proven in spades to prevent and reverse sarcopenia in older adults with hormone deficiencies.

In the case of men with low T, HRT is also a godsend for restoring muscle mass lost over time. Bioidentical testosterone achieves its impressive results through several mechanisms.

Testosterone works to effectively stimulate new muscle formation in the following ways: enhancing gene expression favorable to muscle growth, optimized amino acid utilization (amino acids being the building block of muscle, which is why bodybuilders take amino acid-containing supplements), and stimulating the activity of myoblasts (the precursor cells to skeletal muscle). Without an optimal testosterone level, you can't build muscle – you can tone and keep what you have with your work-outs, but you can't build muscle.

Sexual Performance

Declines in sexual performance and/or desire (libido) are among the most frequent symptoms of hormone deficiencies, commonly experienced by both men and women later in life.

The connective tissue here is that the sex hormones (estrogen/testosterone/progesterone in women and testosterone in men) drive sexual performance and libido. So, when the former drops, so go the latter.

It follows, by way of logic, that replacing the sex hormones to optimal levels in patients with diagnosed deficiencies would help to treat these issues.

In aging men, erectile dysfunction (ED) is incredibly common, and getting more usual by the year for a host of reasons. For evidence, take note the next time you tune into your favorite program just how many commercials on television advertise pharmaceutical solutions in the form of Viagra, Cialis, etc.

While ED pills might temporarily relieve erectile dysfunction and facilitate stiff erections, they unfortunately do not address the underlying cause, which is often a testosterone deficiency. Therefore, their application is quite limited.

Testosterone replacement therapy (TRT), on the other hand, has been shown to reverse ED in men with low T who receive it—without the inconvenient and decidedly unromantic pill-popping planned in advance of an anticipated sexual encounter.

Why not be ready for action whenever the occasion spontaneously arises?

Regarding improvements in libido following TRT, the literature review further concluded that "testosterone therapy has also shown consistent benefit in improving libido in men and women with low testosterone levels at baseline."

The favorable news that testosterone replacement therapy as a remedy for sexual dysfunction and dissatisfaction isn't just for men. You might be surprised to learn that, in addition to supplementing with exogenous estrogen, postmenopausal women may also benefit sexually from adding testosterone into their hormone therapy.

Mental Health

The brain relies on a cornucopia of hormones—in the correct balance—and specialized molecules called neurotransmitters to function optimally.

Indeed, all three of the main sex hormones—estrogen, progesterone, and testosterone—have respective receptor sites (the docking sites on cells designed for interaction with hormones we previously discussed) located prolifically throughout the brain, which indicates their importance to mental and emotional health.

Regions of the brain with sex hormone receptor sites include:

- Prefrontal cortex (involved in decision-making, planning, regulating social behaviors, and other functions by coordinating with other brain regions)
- Cerebral cortex (responsible for higher-level functions such as regulation of emotions, reasoning, memory, language, and personality)
- Cerebellum (regulating muscle function such as movement, coordination, and balance)
- Hippocampus (involved in short-term memory, emotion regulation, and learning)
- Dorsal striatum (closely linked to decision-making processes)
- Hypothalamus (the "command center" for homeostasis, meaning the maintenance of conditions in the body needed to thrive)
- Amygdala (important for regulation of emotions, especially fear and anxiety)

The research on the connection between optimal levels of sex hormones and mental/emotional well-being is clear in its conclusions: they are indispensable to optimal brain health throughout the individual's life span.

The ongoing creation of new synaptic connections—the crucial links between neurons (brain cells) that relay messages throughout the brain—is a must for any anti-aging regimen.

Indeed, memory formation and learning depend entirely on the creation of novel synaptic connections between neurons. The breakdown of synaptic connections is closely linked to the development of neurodegenerative disease, including Alzheimer's and Parkinson's.

The formation of new networks in the brain is a process called "synaptic plasticity"—a fascinating and awe-inspiring concept that has transformed our biological understanding of what the brain is capable of.

It turns out, at a very fundamental physiological level, you *do*—with the right medical and lifestyle strategy—have the power to change your mind.

So, let's put that outdated adage that "you can't teach an old dog new tricks" to bed once and for all. You absolutely can and must continue learning deep into life, and specific medical interventions can help.

If you or a loved one has experienced menopause or testosterone deficiency, you might already know firsthand the depression, anxiety, and other disorders that often accompany a decline in circulating estrogen and/or testosterone.

"Women are at an increased risk of depression and anxiety during perimenopause and the menopausal transition," as explained in research published in Drugs and Aging[18]. "Depressive symptoms experienced in perimenopause are often more severe compared to pre- and post-menopause." Women who have experienced depressive episodes earlier in life are especially at risk of postmenopausal depression, but it can happen to anyone during this transition period.

The same goes for low testosterone: "Several studies indicate that men with low testosterone levels also appear to have more depressive symptoms" per a 2019 meta-analysis of the association between low T and depression published in the Journal of the American Medicine Association Psychiatry [19].

The good news is that we have a documented solution to depression related to declining estrogen/testosterone levels: HRT.

There you have it: whether we're talking about preserving and enhancing memory or keeping your outlook on life bright and vibrant, HRT offers novel solutions where others, like antidepressants, fail to get at the root of the problem.

Cardiovascular (Heart) Health

We've discussed previously the prevalence of sex hormone receptor sites distributed throughout organs and tissues in the body. This phenomenon extends, thankfully, to the heart, the powerhouse organ in your chest that circulates life-giving oxygen and nutrients to the cells and tissues that need them to thrive.

You likely don't need me to tell you that keeping your ticker in tip-top shape is nothing to neglect in terms of achieving a long, healthy life free of the burden of chronic illness; some form of heart disease, statistically, has likely impacted your family in some way.

"Cardiovascular diseases (CVDs) are the leading cause of death globally, taking an estimated 17.9 million lives each year," notes the World Health Organization[20]. "CVDs are a group of disorders of the heart and blood vessels and include coronary heart disease, cerebrovascular disease, rheumatic heart disease and other conditions."

Here, via the Asian Journal of Andrology [21], we have the conclusions of an extensive literature review documenting the relationship between low testosterone levels in aging men and coronary heart disease:

> *"It has now been demonstrated in several large longitudinal cohort studies of men with and without coronary disease that* ***low baseline testosterone is a significant risk marker of*** *increased all-cause and* ***cardiovascular mortality****."*

It's not just men with low T who are at risk of the adverse effects of hormone deficiencies. Heart disease is (almost) an equal-opportunity killer: "In women, physiological levels of estrogen appear protective against atherosclerosis, whereas conditions associated with estrogen deficiency such as early menopause or bilateral oophorectomy are associated with an increased burden of coronary disease," add the study's authors. ("Oophorectomy" is the clinical term that refers to the surgical removal of one or both ovaries, the female sex organs that produce estrogen.)

Enter hormone replacement therapy to save the day.

For men, the clinical evidence of the efficacy of testosterone replacement therapy (TRT) for reducing risk factors associated with heart disease is robust and increasingly indisputable.

TRT reduces heart disease risk through numerous mechanisms, as explained via the Asian Journal of Andrology:

*"**Testosterone supplementation in men with type II diabetes has been shown to reduce total and LDL cholesterol** and lipoprotein a, even in men already established on statin therapy. In studies of elderly and hypogonadal men, testosterone therapy has been associated with improved lipid profiles with reductions in total and LDL cholesterol. Hypotestosteronemia is associated with hypertension and arterial stiffening. There have been several trials of testosterone replacement therapy in eugonadal, hypogonadal and obese men which have observed **impressive reductions in both systolic and diastolic blood pressure** over periods as short as 6 months and for as long as 10 years. Similar beneficial effects of chronic testosterone therapy were demonstrated in **reducing body mass index** in a study of testosterone therapy over a 12-month period. Testosterone therapy induces **increased insulin sensitivity and improved glycemic control** in type II diabetic men. Studies of testosterone therapy have also observed **beneficial modifications in pro- and anti-inflammatory cytokine profiles**."*

To recap, testosterone introduced through therapy in men with low T:

- Tamps down inflammation (a common driver of many chronic illnesses)
- Improves glycemic control (keeping blood sugar in check) and insulin sensitivity (the capacity to transport blood sugar into the cells where it belongs)
- Reduces body fat
- Lowers blood pressure
- Limits LDL cholesterol (the "bad" cholesterol most commonly tied to heart disease)

Women experiencing menopause similarly reap a beneficial preventative effect from bioidentical estrogen supplementation via HRT. Research published in the previously cited Journal of Cancer documents estrogen supplementation's therapeutic impacts on heart disease risks, which exceed, as the authors observe, other clinical interventions such as drugs meant to lower cholesterol levels:

"Initiated in women <60 years of age and/or at or near menopause, ***HRT significantly reduces all-cause mortality and cardiovascular disease (CVD)*** *whereas other primary CVD prevention therapies such as lipid-lowering fail to do so…When initiated in women in their 50s and continued for 5–30 years, HRT reduces all-cause mortality and cost-effectively* ***increases quality adjusted life-years(QALYs)****…*

Menopausal HRT must be considered differently than other medications since ***no other single primary CVD preventive therapy offers diverse systemic-wide benefits****."*

And there you have it: the magic of HRT encompassed in a single succinct phrase in the Journal of Cancer that I wish to impart on my readers: the "systemic-wide benefits" of HRT with bioidentical hormones are second to no other medical intervention because the health improvements delivered to patients are robust and comprehensive across numerous domains—a perfect segue into the next benefit of HRT we'll explore, also connected to heart health: optimal sleep quality.

One thing to remember, when research mentions starting HRT before or after the age of 60, they are basing this on research that was done with Premarin (synthetic), not bioidentical HRT. I am clinically seeing health and life improvements in women I have started on BHRT after the age of 60. Just because you are 60+ years old, doesn't mean there are not significant benefits with BHRT. You may have another 40+ years to live, don't you want them to be fabulous? I do!

Sleep Quality

Proper sleep (7-9 hours per night for most people) is essential for health and longevity. As with most good things in life, it's not just quantity; the quality of the sleep is also paramount. Hormone optimization, fortunately, helps with both.

The odd sleepless night here or there—it happens to the best of us, no matter how we prepare for slumber, so don't beat yourself up counting sheep—won't be damaging enough to do any lasting harm. But chronic sleep deprivation can be devastating for your well-being and put you at greater risk of a slew of chronic conditions ranging from metabolic disorder (diabetes) to cardiovascular disease to neurodegeneration (Alzheimer's or Parkinson's disease, for example).

Vis-à-vis sleep deprivation and hormones, the dilemma we have is a bit of a chicken-or-the-egg situation: does poor sleep cause hormone disturbances, or do hormone imbalances cause poor sleep?

The answer, based on clinical evidence, appears to be *both*. Unhealthy sleep habits negatively impact hormone health, and poor hormone health, in turn, disrupts healthy sleep. It's a bit of a spiral into poor long-term health outcomes and diminished quality of life.

First, let's briefly explore how sleep affects hormone function, via the International Journal of Endocrinology [23]:

> *"The levels of several hormones fluctuate according to the light and dark cycle and are also affected by sleep, feeding, and general behavior.* ***The regulation and metabolism of several hormones are influenced by interactions between the effects of sleep and the intrinsic circadian system****; growth hormone, melatonin, cortisol, leptin, and ghrelin levels are highly correlated with sleep and circadian rhythmicity...* ***Sleep disturbance, which negatively impacts hormonal rhythms and metabolism****, is also associated with obesity, insulin insensitivity, diabetes,* ***hormonal imbalance****, and appetite dysregulation."*

Getting hormones into the optimal range—in addition to important lifestyle adjustments that we'll delve into in an upcoming chapter—is crucial for restoring high-quality sleep and reaping the consequent health benefits.

For patients with a hormone imbalance, HRT can potentially work medical miracles. But, unlike miracles of the sacred sort, there's no prayer or divine intervention necessary. Rather, it's all well-established science.

Similar benefits can be achieved with testosterone replacement therapy—although excessive testosterone levels (such as the result of illegal steroid use) may exacerbate sleep issues, which is why it's critical to undergo TRT with the expert assistance of a hormone healthcare professional to get your T counts into the sweet spot and keep them there.

> *"When low testosterone causes poor sleep, testosterone treatment may improve sleep,"* notes the Sleep Foundation [26].

While it seems odd, I have heard from many patients that after their treatment with me, the very next day "I just had the best night's sleep I have had in years!" At first, I was writing it off to the placebo effect, but then again, you can't placebo sleep! Either you are asleep, or you aren't!

Immune System Function

Your immune system is the brave network of cells, organs, and proteins (including antibodies) that keeps your body safe and protected from invading pathogens like viruses, bacteria, and fungi.

When properly maintained and nourished (including having the right levels of hormones) the immune system is remarkably adept at doing what it's designed to do. Evolution, after all, doesn't make mistakes.

It is only when the body's physiology breaks down that illness ensues.

Biologists divide the human immune system into two complementary components, both of which are equally important:

- The **innate immune system**: this refers to the part of the immune system you are naturally equipped with, designed to respond in *general* terms to all pathogens, whether they have been previously encountered or not
- The **adaptive immune system**: this refers to the part of the immune system that develops over time, learning to recognize pathogens as they are encountered in the environment and developing strategies to neutralize them

Hormones play a vital role in maintaining and promoting a fully functional immune system so that all those pesky little pathogens—which literally surround us at all time as we move through the world—are kept in check, unable to wreak havoc on our health.

Testosterone and estrogen, specifically, exert a bit of a yin and yang effect on immune system modulation.

This dynamic illustrates the importance of keeping both sex hormones in the proper balance. The dangers of an underactive (suppressed) immune system (associated with excessive testosterone relative to estrogen) are obvious: you're going to get sick more easily. But the less obvious dangers of an overactive immune system (potentially triggered by excessive estrogen relative to testosterone) are just as great.

(The immune-suppressing effects of testosterone vs. immune-enhancing effects of estrogen also explain why men are more vulnerable to infectious disease while women statistically have a higher proportion of autoimmune disease, which we'll get into coming up.)

As always, the devil is in the details, which is why it's important—and I'll continue to emphasize this—to work with a seasoned hormone expert to get the exact ratios and levels of the hormones right. The optimal dose of testosterone replacement therapy (TRT) needs to be determined to strike the fine balance in varied indications

The same results regarding hormone optimization and improved outcomes in forms of acute infections in addition to COVID-19 are legion, which I will spare here for the sake of brevity. Suffice it to say the clinical evidence is conclusive: healthy hormone levels mean a healthier immune system.

Let's segue here into the previously mentioned scourge of autoimmune disease in our modern world, a term that refers to a malfunction of the adaptive immune system in which the mechanisms of the immune system are unleashed on your healthy, normal tissues, at which time disease ensues ("auto" meaning "self," hence "self"-attacking immune response).

Common examples of autoimmune disease plaguing our modern world include:

- Rheumatoid arthritis
- Multiple sclerosis
- Graves' disease
- Type 1 diabetes
- Celiac disease
- Inflammatory bowel disease
- Lupus
- Hashimoto's thyroiditis

Altogether, these illnesses cut short the lives of *millions* of Americans every year. The "lucky" ones merely experience drastic reductions in their quality of life.

In the face of all of this, modern medicine has until now been largely helpless to stem the increasing rates of autoimmune disease, due in no small part to the incredible complexity of the immune system, which we in the medical community have just begun to fully understand at a molecular level.

That said, it is my clinical experience that, in the right contexts, HRT can help manage and treat autoimmune disease that does not otherwise respond to conventional treatments.

For instance, "in rheumatoid arthritis, HRT does not appear to be associated with an increased risk of disease flare and may actually improve disease activity," per a 2009 research paper published in the medical journal Climacteric [30].

"We strongly recommend estrogen replacement therapy to prevent postmenopausal osteoporosis in women with rheumatoid arthritis. Younger women with rheumatoid arthritis can undergo pregnancy or use estrogen-containing contraceptives," add the researchers of a literature review published in the Cleveland Clinic Journal of Medicine [31].

Hormone optimization, let's be clear, is by no means the only answer—a silver bullet, if you will—to solving our autoimmunity crisis, but hormone imbalance is *absolutely* an underappreciated and undertreated factor in autoimmune disease that must be addressed to overcome it.

PTSD

In popular culture, post-traumatic stress disorder (commonly abbreviated using the acronym PTSD) is most associated with soldiers returning home from combat. (Historically, PTSD was called "shell shock.") If you are already familiar with the term, trauma induced by war is likely the context. I treat many first responders that suffer from PTSD just imagine the horrible sights they see daily. One of my fire fighter patients says she remembers the smell of the first burning body she had to rescue. May God bless her.

PTSD may tragically afflict soldiers, first responders, and others who have lived through the horrors of war and life. However, combat veterans are by no stretch of the imagination the only individuals susceptible to PTSD, which can affect anyone at any age, including survivors of:

- physical assault
- sexual assault
- emotional/psychological abuse
- domestic abuse
- natural disasters
- car accidents
- falls
- any other form of physical trauma
- bullying

...and more.

PTSD is far more common than you might believe. The American Psychiatric Association [32] explains the prevalence of PTSD in the United States and how it manifests clinically:

> ***"PTSD affects approximately 3.5 percent of U.S. adults every year...*** *An estimate [sic]* ***one in 11 people will be diagnosed with***

> ***PTSD in their lifetime.*** *Women are twice as likely as men to have PTSD...*
>
> **People with PTSD have intense, disturbing thoughts and feelings related to their experience that last long after the traumatic event has ended.** *They may relive the event through flashbacks or nightmares;* **they may feel sadness, fear or anger; and they may feel detached or estranged from other people.** *People with PTSD may avoid situations or people that remind them of the traumatic event, and* ***they may have strong negative reactions to something as ordinary as a loud noise or an accidental touch.***"

But even the figures presented above may be under-representative of the true disease burden, as many individuals affected by PTSD may not know they have it and may not receive a diagnosis, thus unnecessarily extending their suffering and limiting public awareness of this debilitating condition.

(If you have noticed any of these symptoms in yourself or a loved one, especially if there is a potentially traumatic event in the past that they might be tied to, it's worth exploring the possibility of PTSD with a qualified professional.)

The good news is that: a) awareness of PTSD both in the population at large and among healthcare professionals has expanded greatly in the past several years and; b) there are many potential treatments.

Treatments with clinical backing to treat PTSD include:

- Various forms of psychotherapy, including cognitive behavioral therapy and eye movement desensitization and reprocessing (EMDR)
- Medication
- Social support groups
- Hormone replacement therapy

On the last score, let's consider the findings of an extensive literature review via the medical journal Biological Psychiatry [33] in the context, specifically, of women affected by PTSD and the potential relief gained through HRT with estrogen:

> *"**The association between low estrogen and fear extinction has great clinical significance,** as they suggest that **elevating estrogen levels in some patients may prove beneficial in rescuing extinction deficits observed in PTSD*.** A recent proof-of-concept study found that administration of synthetic estrogen to normally cycling healthy volunteers increased extinction recall after fear extinction training (87). Due to the fact that clinical exposure therapy recruits neural learning mechanisms that mediate conditioned fear extinction, the adjuvant use of estrogen could facilitate therapeutic effects in fewer sessions…*
>
> *Similar studies have found that **estradiol administration significantly alleviated symptoms of depression in peri-menopausal women.** A recent naturalistic study compared sexual assault victims who either received or declined estrogen-based emergency contraceptives immediately after the assault and found that those who took estrogen had significantly lower PTSD symptoms 6 months later. **The studies reviewed here support the use of estrogen as an individualized treatment strategy in women with PTSD.**"*

*"Fear extinction" is the clinical term that refers to "unlearning" the irrational fear responses to any given trigger (as classic examples, loud noises or unexpected touch) characteristic of PTSD—achieving fear extinction being a fundamental component of psychotherapeutic approaches to treating the disorder.

Healthier testosterone levels in both men *and* women, similarly, are linked to a reduced risk of developing PTSD, as well as to the facilitation of improved therapeutic outcomes to treat PTSD.

While we know HRT is not going to cure PTSD, it may help with many of the symptoms such as anxiety, depression, sleep issues, mood swings, relationships, and fatigue. I had a first responder that I treated the day after she was released from the hospital after a suicide attempt. When I saw her at her follow-up visit, she cried and hugged me and told me that I was her angel–saying I had saved her life! Wow.

Inflammation

By now I've alluded to the health threat posed by inflammation, specifically chronic inflammation, a couple of times, but it deserves a section all its own for reasons I'll explain now.

You might be familiar with inflammation in the context of an injury: you stub your toe and, as a result, it gets red and swollen. Ouch!

That type of inflammation—called *acute* inflammation—is healthy and normal, as it allows the body to begin the repair process. You need a healthy inflammatory response in the unfortunate toe-stubbing incident now and again to get the ball rolling on healing.

It's called "acute" inflammation because it's intended to be short in duration and disappear once it's done its job, which is helping your damaged cells and tissues heal.

Contrast normal and healthy acute inflammation with an absolute killer: *chronic* inflammation—meaning long-lasting without any resolution.

What we see indicated in the literature and what I see firsthand in my practice is that chronic inflammation is implicated in virtually every form of chronic illness known to man, as explained via research from the journal Nature Medicine [35]:

> *"Although intermittent increases in inflammation are critical for survival during physical injury and infection, recent research has revealed that certain social, environmental and lifestyle factors can promote* ***systemic chronic inflammation (SCI)*** *that* ***can****, in turn,* ***lead to several diseases*** *that collectively represent the leading causes of disability and mortality worldwide,* ***such as cardiovascular disease, cancer, diabetes mellitus, chronic kidney***

disease, non-alcoholic fatty liver disease and autoimmune and neurodegenerative disorders."

Cancers, heart disease, autoimmune diseases like MS, neurodegenerative diseases like Alzheimer's... what these diverse but universally devastating conditions have in common is that they all heavily feature an aspect of untreated chronic inflammation.

The good news is that chronic inflammation is both diagnosable and treatable.

At LowTE Florida, we have several tests at our disposal that we can run to determine your levels of chronic inflammation. Here is a handful of the handiest markers of inflammation:

- **High-sensitivity C-reactive protein** (hs-CRP). CRP is a protein synthesized in the liver in reaction to chronic inflammation. As chronic inflammation levels increase, so do CRP levels.
- **Erythrocyte sedimentation rate** (ESR). The purpose of the ESR test is to gauge how quickly red blood cells settle at the bottom of an upright test tube. Chronic inflammation results in greater protein concentration in the blood, which causes red blood cells to settle faster.

- **Homocysteine** Since inflammation promotes cell proliferation at the expense of excess vitamins leading to hyperhomocysteinemia, therefore, homocysteine can be used as a marker of inflammation to indicate the presence of inflammation.

- **Fibrinogen** is the name of a protein the liver produces to facilitate blood clots to slow and stop bleeding. While a certain amount of fibrinogen is critical for good health, when chronic inflammation is abnormally high, so are fibrinogen levels.

While these tests are not included in our initial laboratory panel at LowTE Florida (some require specialized handling we are unable provide) you can always ask us to write you a prescription you can take to a commercial lab to assess your inflammation.

If we determine through clinical testing and other methods of evaluation that you are experiencing chronic inflammation, there are many proven remedies available to us at LowTE Florida, including bioidentical hormone replacement therapy.

Multiple studies have consistently demonstrated sex hormones' mediating effects on chronic inflammation, for example the following two-year trial regarding the benefits of estrogen therapy on inflammatory markers from the medical journal Arthritis Research & Therapy [36]:

> *"Is there any evidence that HRT has beneficial effects on established [rheumatoid arthritis]?* ***We recently completed a 2-year controlled, randomized and prospective trial*** *comparing calcium/vitamin D3 + HRT and calcium/vitamin D3 alone in patients with long-lasting [rheumatoid arthritis*__*].*__ ***The outcome clearly showed that the HRT-treated patients responded with a significant decrease in*** *Disease Activity Score 28 and* ***laboratory signs of inflammation*** *(sedimentation rate and hemoglobin), an increase in bone mineral density and less progression of radiographic joint destruction compared with controls."*

And, for men, here's what bioidentical testosterone therapy can do for chronic inflammation: the evidence shows that markers of chronic inflammation increase in men with low T and decrease once testosterone is introduced through therapy, as documented by way of The Aging Male [37]:

> ***"Low testosterone levels are found to be associated with an increased in metabolic risk and systematic inflammation****. Since adipose tissue is a source of inflammatory cytokines, testosterone may regulate inflammation by acting on adipose tissue.* ***This review aimed to explore the role of testosterone in inflammation*** *and its mechanism of action. Both animal studies and human studies showed* ***that (1) testosterone deficiency was associated with an increase in pro-inflammatory cytokines; (2) testosterone substitution reduced pro-inflammatory cytokines****. The suppression*

of inflammation by testosterone were observed in patients with coronary artery disease, prostate cancer and diabetes mellitus through the increase in anti-inflammatory cytokines (IL-10) and the decrease in pro-inflammatory cytokines (IL-1β, IL-6, and TNF-α)"

Bringing It Home

We've covered a lot of ground in the preceding pages documenting the proven benefits of hormone therapy for healing and reversing health conditions ranging from depression to muscle loss to immune system dysfunction. I'm always excited to serve as the bearer of good news vis-à-vis the benefits of BHRT with current and prospective patients, so many thanks for coming along for the ride!

The key takeaway I'd like to emphasize here, which I always aim to impart to all my patients, is that there is literally no aspect of health that is untouched by hormones. As such, there is no achieving a long-term, sustainable, optimal state of wellness without addressing hormones.

However, not all hormones used in therapy are created equal. Coming up, we'll explore the distinctions you need to understand between bioidentical hormones (the ones I use in my clinical practice for reasons we'll delve into), and synthetic hormones used previously.

References

[1] Campbell, M., Jialal, I. (2022). Physiology, Endocrine Hormones. StatPearls https://www.ncbi.nlm.nih.gov/books/NBK538498/

[2] Teoli, D., Bhardwaj, A. (2023). StatPearls. https://www.ncbi.nlm.nih.gov/books/NBK536962/

[3] Welton, A., Vickers, M., et al. (2008). Health related quality of life after combined hormone replacement therapy: randomized controlled trial. British Medical Journal. https://www.ncbi.nlm.nih.gov/pmc/articles/PMC2518695/

[4] Kent, A. (2008). Hormone Replacement Therapy and Quality of Life. Reviews in Obstetrics and Gynecology. https://www.ncbi.nlm.nih.gov/pmc/articles/PMC2621049

[5] Tokish, J., DeRosa, D. (2014). Pharmacologic Approaches to the Aging Athlete. Sports Health. https://www.ncbi.nlm.nih.gov/pmc/articles/PMC3874227/

[6] Sipila, S., Taaffe, D., et al. (2001). Effects of hormone replacement therapy and high-impact physical exercise on skeletal muscle in post-menopausal women: a randomized placebo-controlled study. Clinical Science (London). https://pubmed.ncbi.nlm.nih.gov/11473488/

[7] Walston, J. (2012). "Sarcopenia in older adults." Current Opinion in Rheumatology. https://www.ncbi.nlm.nih.gov/pmc/articles/PMC4066461/

[8] Shin, M., Jeon, Y., et al. (2018). Testosterone and Sarcopenia. The World Journal of Men's Health. https://www.ncbi.nlm.nih.gov/pmc/articles/PMC6119844/

[9] Kim, S. and Kim, R. (2020). The association between hormone therapy and sarcopenia in postmenopausal women: the Korea National Health and Nutrition Examination Survey, 2008-2011. Menopause. https://www.ncbi.nlm.nih.gov/pmc/articles/PMC7188056/

[10] Junnila, R., List, E., et al. (2013). The GH/IGF-1 axis in ageing and longevity. Nature Reviews Endocrinology. https://www.ncbi.nlm.nih.gov/pmc/articles/PMC4074016/

[11] Rizk, P., Kohn, T., et al. (2017). Testosterone Therapy Improves Erectile Function and Libido in Hypogonadal Men. Current Opinion in Urology. https://www.ncbi.nlm.nih.gov/pmc/articles/PMC5649360/

[12] Shifren, J., Davis, S. (2006). Testosterone patch for the treatment of hypoactive sexual desire disorder in naturally menopausal women: results from the INTIMATE NM1 Study. Menopause. https://pubmed.ncbi.nlm.nih.gov/16932240/

[13] Almey, A., Milner, T., et al. (2015). Estrogen receptors in the central nervous system and their implication for dopamine-dependent cognition in females. Hormones and Behavior. https://www.ncbi.nlm.nih.gov/pmc/articles/PMC4820286/

[14] Ramirez, A., Arbuckle, M. (2016). Synaptic Plasticity: The Role of Learning and Unlearning in Addiction and Beyond. Biological Psychiatry. https://www.ncbi.nlm.nih.gov/pmc/articles/PMC5347979/

[15] Ming, G. and Song, H. (2011). Adult Neurogenesis in the Mammalian Brain: Significant Answers and Significant Questions. Neuron. https://www.ncbi.nlm.nih.gov/pmc/articles/PMC3106107/

[16] Maioli, S., Leander, K. (2021). Estrogen receptors and the aging brain. Essays in Biochemistry. https://www.ncbi.nlm.nih.gov/pmc/articles/PMC8628183/

[17] Kuwahara, M., Nicholson, K., et al. (2021). Androgen Effects on Neural Plasticity. Androgens: Clinical Research and Therapeutics. https://www.ncbi.nlm.nih.gov/pmc/articles/PMC8744448/

[18] Herson, M., Kulkarni, J. (2022). Hormonal Agents for the Treatment of Depression Associated with the Menopause. Drugs and Aging. https://www.ncbi.nlm.nih.gov/pmc/articles/PMC9355926/

[19] Walthier, A., Breidensstein, J., et al. (2019). Association of Testosterone Treatment With Alleviation of Depressive Symptoms in Men. Journal of

the American Medicine Association Psychiatry. https://www.ncbi.nlm.nih.gov/pmc/articles/PMC6583468/

[20] World Health Organization. (n.d.) Cardiovascular diseases. https://www.who.int/health-topics/cardiovascular-diseases#tab=tab_1

[21] Morris, P., Channer, K. (2012). Testosterone and cardiovascular disease in men. Asian Journal of Andrology. https://www.ncbi.nlm.nih.gov/pmc/articles/PMC3720171/

[22] Hodis, H., Mack, W. (2022). Menopausal Hormone Replacement Therapy and Reduction of All-Cause Mortality and Cardiovascular Disease: It's About Time and Timing. Journal of Cancer. https://www.ncbi.nlm.nih.gov/pmc/articles/PMC9178928/

[23] Kim, T., Jeong, J., et al. (2015). The Impact of Sleep and Circadian Disturbance on Hormones and Metabolism. International Journal of Endocrinology. https://www.ncbi.nlm.nih.gov/pmc/articles/PMC4377487/

[24] Wittert, G. (2014). The relationship between sleep disorders and testosterone in men. Asian Journal of Andrology. https://www.ncbi.nlm.nih.gov/pmc/articles/PMC3955336/

[25] Polo-Kantola, P., Errkola, R. (1998). When does estrogen replacement therapy improve sleep quality? American Journal of Obstetrics and Gynecology. https://pubmed.ncbi.nlm.nih.gov/9609575

[26] Suni, E., Adavadkar, P. (2023). How Does Testosterone Affect Sleep? Sleep Foundation https://www.sleepfoundation.org/physical-health/sleep-and-testosterone

[27] Taneja, V. (2018). Sex Hormones Determine Immune Response. Frontiers in Immunology. https://www.ncbi.nlm.nih.gov/pmc/articles/PMC6119719/

[28] Averyanova, M., Vishnyakova, P. (2022). Sex hormones and immune system: Menopausal hormone therapy in the context of COVID-19 pandemic. Frontiers in Immunology. https://www.ncbi.nlm.nih.gov/pmc/articles/PMC9379861/

[29] Hussain, A., Hussain, F. (2020). Role of testosterone in COVID-19 patients—A double-edged sword? Medical Hypotheses. https://www.ncbi.nlm.nih.gov/pmc/articles/PMC7494488/

[30] Holroyd, C., Edwards, C. (2009). The effects of hormone replacement therapy on autoimmune disease: rheumatoid arthritis and systemic lupus erythematosus. Climacteric. https://pubmed.ncbi.nlm.nih.gov/19591008/

[31] Van Vollenhoven, R. (1994). Estrogen, progesterone, and testosterone: can they be used to treat autoimmune diseases? Cleveland Clinic Journal of Medicine. https://pubmed.ncbi.nlm.nih.gov/7923746/

[32] American Psychiatric Association. (n.d.) What is Posttraumatic Stress Disorder (PTSD)? https://www.psychiatry.org/patients-families/ptsd/what-is-ptsd

[33] Glover, E., Jovanovic, T., et al. (2015). Estrogen and Extinction of Fear Memories: Implications for Posttraumatic Stress Disorder Treatment. Biological Psychiatry. https://www.ncbi.nlm.nih.gov/pmc/articles/PMC4757430/

[34] Krine, E., Held, U., et al. Sex hormones and cortisol during experimental trauma memory consolidation: Prospective association with intrusive memories. European Journal of Psychotraumatology. https://www.ncbi.nlm.nih.gov/pmc/articles/PMC8979510/

[35] Furman, D., Campisi, J., et al. (2019). Chronic inflammation in the etiology of disease across the life span. Nature Medicine. https://www.ncbi.nlm.nih.gov/pmc/articles/PMC7147972/

[36] Caristen, H., D'Elia, H., et al. (2004). Menopause and hormone replacement therapy: effects on the immune system, arthritis and bone. Arthritis Research & Therapy. https://www.ncbi.nlm.nih.gov/pmc/articles/PMC2833501/

[37] Mohamad, M., Wong, S., et al. (2019). The relationship between circulating testosterone and inflammatory cytokines in men. The Aging Male. https://pubmed.ncbi.nlm.nih.gov/29925283/

Chapter IV
The History of Hormone Replacement Therapy

We established in the previous chapter that modern sick care, unfortunately, far too often, neglects hormone care (and other critical aspects of healthcare that we'll explore coming up). This deficiency is much to the detriment of patients, as hormone care is a central, critical pillar of an effective wellness-enhancing, anti-aging strategy.

In the upcoming chapters, we're going to focus on what hormones do and why their proper function is nothing short of *indispensable* to achieving your best health.

The bottom line is: if you're not optimizing your hormones, especially later in life, you're not optimizing your health.

But before we get to that, we need to briefly establish the storied, meandering—and sometimes strange—history of hormone replacement therapy (HRT).

We're going to explore how it fell out of fashion over two decades ago due to faulty research and misleading media reporting, and how anti-aging medical practitioners like me have diligently revived the science and art of hormone optimization—even when we were lost in the weeds, cast to the fringes of the profession.

The use of bioidentical hormones is not new. Notably, my own family has contributed to this field. My Great Uncle Frederick Conrad Koch, a pioneering biochemist and endocrinologist, made significant strides in understanding male sex hormones and testicular function.

Born in Chicago, Illinois, in 1876, Uncle Fred graduated from the University of Illinois in 1899 and went on to affiliate with the University of Chicago from 1912 to 1941, serving as chairman of the department of biochemistry from 1936 to 1941. His work primarily focused on male sex hormones and testicular function, laying crucial groundwork for modern hormone research.

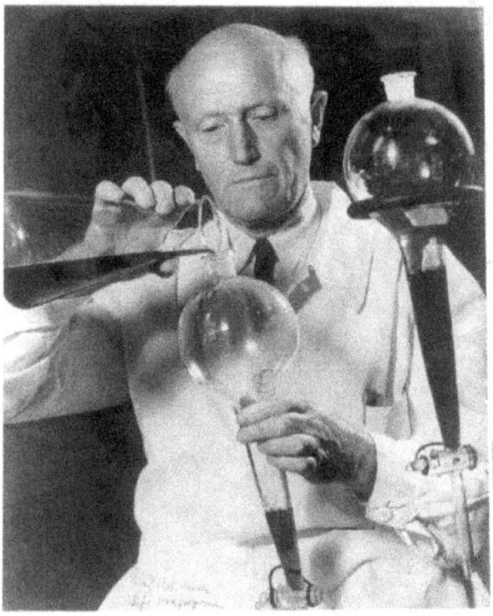

Uncle Fred's achievements were recognized by the Endocrine Society, which established the Fred Conrad Koch Lifetime Achievement Award in 1957 – the society's highest honor. He served as the 19th president of the Endocrine Society and later became director of biomedical research at Armour® and Company.

A notable testament to his work is the picture featured in Life Magazine, showcasing his dedication to advancing our understanding of hormones and thyroid function. This legacy inspires me to continue pushing the boundaries of hormone optimization.

The brief history of HRT—the term that refers to the strategic supplementation of exogenous (meaning "from outside the body") hormones to make up for deficits often experienced by older patients—begins in the 1930s. Bioidentical hormones have been used in the United States for over 85 years. the first research study I can find is from 1939. In 1942, the first-ever FDA-approved synthetic estrogen formulation called Premarin®, a "conjugated estrogen" derived from pregnant horse urine, to treat hot flashes was brought to market [1]. Over time, synthetic estrogen won FDA approval to treat a variety of other conditions associated with aging and hormone deficits, including osteoporosis—the progressive weakening of the bones that is a leading cause of disability among older patients, especially women.

Books like the 1966 seminal treatise on the topic, "Feminine Forever," popularized HRT as a treatment for menopause, a technique that was ushered into mainstream medicine on the coattails of the first and second-wave feminist movements of the period.

Suddenly, the collective social realization occurred that menopause need no longer be a painful, inevitable phase of life to be suffered in silence by women. Finally, there was hope for relief!

Naturally, women gravitated to HRT by the millions, and it steadily became increasingly common as a first-resort treatment for menopause symptoms as its benefits were manifest and undeniable.

The human body is infinitely complex (especially in comparison to our limited understanding of it), as is the hormone system. Our approach to healthcare must be equally nuanced and grounded in humility and a willingness to embrace new information as it becomes available.

Taking the 10,000 ft. above sea level view is what I do at LowTE Florida, as do all expert anti-aging medicine practitioners. **Optimizing the level of any given single hormone is no more important than optimizing the balance of hormones in relation to one another.**

In the meanwhile, the popularity of HRT continued to grow as women experienced the irrefutable benefits firsthand, proving the adage true: nothing trumps personal experience. The HRT genie can only be kept in the bottle for so long when the often-transformative benefits are so evident to the men and women who receive it and the clinical providers who deliver it.

Finally, HRT looked to be on the cusp of breaking permanently into mainstream medicine once and for all when, in 2002, a damning yet poorly designed study threw cold water, once again, on our practice.

The study—called the Women's Health Initiative (WHI)—was mammoth in its scale, involving over 100,000 women, spanning 15 years, and costing more than $260 million. Its purpose? To study the health impacts of menopause on postmenopausal women with the aim of developing more ideal treatment protocols.

"But **in June 2002**, word started spreading that **one arm of the trial** in which women were given a combination of estrogen and progestin, a synthetic form of progesterone **had been stopped prematurely**," according to The New York Times [4] in a retrospective post-mortem on the study published in February 2023. "Jaques Rossouw, **an epidemiologist who was the acting director of the W.H.I., told the gathered press that the study had found both adverse effects and benefits of hormone therapy**, but that 'the adverse effects outweigh and outnumber the benefits.'"

"Researchers and news anchors presented the data in a way that caused panic," The New York Times adds.

This was huge—and hugely detrimental—publicity for the HRT industry, the medical practitioners who had made their careers out of optimizing hormones in postmenopausal women and, most devastatingly, the millions of aging female patients themselves who had, by the WHI's own admission, experienced substantial benefits from treatment with supplemental estrogen.

So, what did the WHI researchers get wrong, and what can we learn from this travesty as clinicians and laypeople learning to read clinical literature through a clinical lens? The New York Times summarizes:

> *"The study itself was designed with what would come to be seen as a major flaw. W.H.I. researchers wanted to be able to measure health outcomes how many women ended up having strokes, heart attacks or cancer but those ailments may not show up until women are in their 70s or 80s. The study was scheduled to run for only 8½ years. So,* ***they weighted the participants toward women who were already 60 or older****. That choice meant that* ***women in their 50s, who tended to be healthier and have more menopausal symptoms, were underrepresented in the study****. At the news conference, Rossouw started out by saying that the findings had 'broad applicability,' emphasizing that the trial found no difference in risk by age.* ***It would be years before researchers appreciated just how wrong that was****…*

[Stephanie] Faubion, who is also the medical director of the North American Menopause Society (NAMS), an association of menopause specialists, says the first question patients usually ask her is about breast-cancer risk. She explains that ***in the W.H.I. trial, women who were given a combination of estrogen and progestin saw an increased risk emerge only after five years on hormones*** *and* ***even after 20 years, the mortality rate of women who took those hormones was no higher than that of the control group****...*

When [chief of the division of preventive medicine at Brigham and Women's Hospital JoAnn] Manson, along with [epidemiologist Jaques] Rossouw, did a reanalysis of the W.H.I. findings, she found that ***women under 60 in the trial had no elevated risk of heart disease****."*

So, to wrap up, the major flaws of the landmark WHI study were:

- Recruiting participants who were already over 60, meaning they were less likely to benefit from synthetic HRT, having on average already gone through menopause, and were more likely to experience negative health events like heart attacks, strokes, and cancer that posed much less risk for younger women who were more likely to benefit from synthetic or even better, bioidentical HRT
- Not differentiating between HRT involving estrogen alone and estrogen *in combination with the complementary hormone progestin* (the latter substantially resulting in lower adverse outcomes to the extent of rendering the risk negligible).
- Not recognizing the difference between bioidentical HRT and synthetic—what was bad about synthetic was good with bioidentical! Apples and oranges but the media, still today, doesn't report if the studies they are talking about are with synthetic or bioidentical hormones! Very frustrating!

Basically, they did everything wrong. They used synthetic hormones, they didn't personalize the dosing (everyone got the same doses), and they used the worst delivery system (oral pills).

Alas, shortcomings notwithstanding, the damage had been done with the 2002 melodrama; within just seven years of the WHI debacle, insurance claims for HRT had dropped by more than 70%. One doctor at a major hospital described it as "the most dramatic sea change in clinical medicine that [they had] ever seen."

Since then, fortunately, the practice of HRT—particularly for the treatment of menopause but also in the form of testosterone replacement therapy (TRT) for men with low T and other applications—has bounced back admirably.

A 2016 analysis titled "Menopause Management Getting Clinical Care Back on Track," [5] authored by the JoAnn Manson, published in the prestigious New England Journal of Medicine, for instance, has gone a long way to right the wrongs from the 2002 WHI study by placing its findings in the proper context and injecting scientific rigor into its analysis.

The New York Times concludes its treatise on the WHI saga with a dizzying (but, as we will see coming up, still incomplete) overview of the since-documented benefits of estrogen therapy for menopausal women:

> *"Researchers also now have a better appreciation of the benefits of hormone therapy. Even at the time that the W.H.I. findings were released, the data showed at least one clear improvement resulting from hormone therapy: Women had 24 percent fewer fractures. Since then, other positive results have emerged. The incidence of diabetes, for instance, was found to be 20 percent lower in women who took hormones, compared with those who took a placebo. In the W.H.I. trial, women who had hysterectomies30 percent of American women by age 60were given estrogen alone because they did not need progesterone to protect them from endometrial cancer, and that group had lower*

rates of breast cancer than the placebo group... Positive reports about hormone therapy for women in their 50s started emerging as early as 2003, and they have never really slowed."

In addition to faulty studies like the 2002 WHI leading to improper extrapolations that trigger a media avalanche of negative stories, the vital importance of hormones to long-term wellness is poorly understood by many practitioners of mainstream medicine for many other reasons.

Perhaps the most important of these is that **the curricula used in medical schools** from coast to coast **do not sufficiently focus on hormones or the hormone system** (called the "endocrine system" in clinical literature).

Here's a common scenario that you may have experienced yourself at some point:

- Feeling unwell, you visit your primary care doctor or an urgent care facility. Maybe the issue is a chronic headache; maybe it's lack of energy; maybe it's spiraling depression.
- You explain your symptoms to your doctor.
- Your healthcare provider listens while staring into their computer—perhaps for just a minute or two—and *possibly* asks a follow-up question or two and *possibly* orders a basic blood panel or other lab exam (often with no testing for hormones). Just as likely, they simply absorb your complaints with minimal inquiry on their part.
- Your provider then offers a quick fix that does not address the underlying cause of your state of disease. (For instance, he or she might prescribe an SSRI antidepressant—an extremely common drug with numerous side effects and a questionable mechanism of action that may have effects on some patients but not others—for the resolution of mental health symptoms without fixing the hormonal trigger.)
- You return to your daily life, you experience no or limited relief, and you continue to needlessly suffer in your quality of life with no real idea of what's going on in your physiology or how to change it for the better.

This isn't to say, again, that many doctors, nurses, and other hands-on healthcare providers don't mean well. These are, by and large, individuals who devoted their lives for the noblest of reasons to helping patients live better and longer.

Rather than malice or negligence, there might be many reasons far too many providers fail to address hormones in their diagnostic processes—which, to emphasize once again, very frequently are the root cause of any given health issue. These deficits might include lack of knowledge on the topic, lack of resources, lack of time to fully investigate each patient's case, or all the above.

The widespread oversight of hormones in clinical care is not just my subjective opinion based on years of practice myself, during which I have interacted with thousands of patients and heard the same stories over and over. In addition to the testimonials of patients, we also have a wealth of quantitative data to rely on.

Let's consider, for instance, the results of a 2019 survey of medical school residents published in the medical journal Mayo Clinic Proceedings [6], which set out to "to evaluate the knowledge of and nature of training for menopause management in postgraduate residents."

Here is an excerpt of the findings:

> *"Of the 703 surveys sent, a total of 183 residents representing 20 US residency programs responded (26.0% response rate). Most trainees were between 26 and 30 years of age (133 of 172 [77.3%]), female (114 of 173 [65.9%]), and believed it was important or very important to be trained to manage menopause (165 of 176 [93.8%]).* ***Although most respondents answered some of the menopause competency questions correctly, important gaps were identified****. Of 183 participants, 63* ***(34.4%) indicated they would not offer HT to a symptomatic, newly menopausal woman without contraindications****, and only 71 (38.7%) indicated they would prescribe HT until the natural age of menopause to a*

prematurely menopausal woman. Of 177 respondents, 36 (20.3%) reported not receiving any menopause lectures during residency, and ***only*** *12 of 177* ***(6.8%) reported feeling adequately prepared to manage women experiencing menopause****."*

Let that sink in just 6.8% of medical school residents reported feeling "adequately prepared" to help women going through menopause can be described as nothing except an abject failure of our training institutions to equip our nurses and doctors with the tools and knowledge they need to help their patients fully heal from a condition—menopause—that all women will experience at some point in the aging process.

The basic problem with large medical institutions like hospital systems and specialty organizations is they often adhere to a rigid set of protocols that do not allow flexibility and do not encourage practitioners to think "outside of the box" when it comes to delivering care. The result is that if HRT isn't a standard prescribed protocol, it's not going to be offered to patients. And if the providers aren't specifically educated in the administration of hormone care, they won't even be aware of what potential relief they're denying their patients.

Many patients tell me that their healthcare providers won't even test their blood for hormones. My thinking is that they aren't testing them because they don't know how to analyze the lab test results and optimize their hormones. This is my expertise. I've got this!

My hope is that the picture I've painted here is clear: the burden is on all of us, providers and patients alike, to educate ourselves about the vital role that hormones play in long-term health and adjust our therapeutic approaches accordingly. This work is central to my mission at LowTE Florida, and the reason I have compiled the information contained in these pages.

Thankfully, due to that work that I and hundreds, if not thousands, of my colleagues have done over the intervening decades to prove the worth of hormone optimization, the paradigm has finally begun to shift in our favor.

One of the catalyzing factors in the renewal of interest in hormones is the unfortunate prevalence of synthetic, hormone-disrupting chemicals (sometimes called "endocrine disruptors") in the modern environment that have driven an increase in hormone-related disorders, as explained in a 2005 publication from EMBO Reports [10]:

> *"In addition to purely scientific advances, the study of hormones has led to enormous benefits to human health, social and economic progress, such as contraception, in vitro fertilization (IVF) and recombinant human hormones. More recently,* ***the topic of hormones*** *and hormonally regulated metabolism and development* ***has also found interest among public health experts*** *and the larger public,* ***after concerned scientists in the USA hypothesized that various man-made chemicals could interfere with the hormonal system to cause a wide range of diseases and disorders.*** *"*

Such endocrine disruptors are widespread and found in many consumer products, such as detergents, plastic bottles, food products, and even the air and water supply! Examples of these toxic compounds include phthalates, bisphenol A (an estrogen mimicker), dioxins, and more.

Coming up in a later chapter, we'll explore strategies that you can use in conjunction with HRT to minimize your exposure to these harmful chemicals and keep your hormone system in top form.

References

[1] Cagnacci, A., Venier, M. (2019). The controversial history of Hormone Replacement therapy. Medicina (Kaunas, Lithuania). https://www.ncbi.nlm.nih.gov/pmc/articles/PMC6780820/

[2] Smith D.C., et al. (1975.) Association of exogenous estrogen and endogenous carcinoma. New England Journal of Medicine. https://pubmed.ncbi.nlm.nih.gov/1186789/

[3] Woodruff, J., et al. (1994). Incidence of endometrial hyperplasia in postmenopausal women taking. American Journal of Obstetrics and Gynecology. https://www.ajog.org/article/S0002-9378(94)70129-6/fulltext

[4] Dominus, S. (2023). Women have been misled about menopause. The New York Times. https://www.nytimes.com/2023/02/01/magazine/menopause-hot-flashes-hormone-therapy.html

[5] Manson, J. and Kaunitz, A. (2016). Menopause Management—getting clinical care back on Track. New England Journal of Medicine. https://www.nejm.org/doi/full/10.1056/NEJMp1514242

[6] Kling, J., MacLaughlin, M., et al. (2019). Menopause Management Knowledge in postgraduate family medicine, Internal Medicine, and obstetrics and gynecology residents: A cross-sectional survey. Mayo Clinic proceedings. https://pubmed.ncbi.nlm.nih.gov/30711122/

[7] Berga, S., Garovic, V. (2020). Barriers to the care of menopausal women. Mayo Clinic proceedings. https://www.ncbi.nlm.nih.gov/pmc/articles/PMC6597249/

[8] Aljumah, R., Phillips, S., et al. (2023). An online survey of postmenopausal women to determine their attitudes and knowledge of the menopause. Post Reproductive Health. https://journals.sagepub.com/doi/10.1177/20533691231166543

[9] Khan, S., Kapoor, E., et al. (2023). Vasomotor Symptoms During Menopause: A Practical Guide on Current Treatments and Future Perspectives. International Journal of Women's Health. https://www.ncbi.nlm.nih.gov/pmc/articles/PMC9938702/

[10] Tata, J. R. (2005). One Hundred Years of hormones. EMBO reports. https://www.ncbi.nlm.nih.gov/pmc/articles/PMC1369102/

Chapter V

What Are *Bioidentical Hormones* and How Do They Supercharge Your Health?

Now that we've established the importance of hormone optimization for long-term health, longevity and quality of life, we're finally getting down to brass tacks, ladies and gentlemen: bioidentical hormones, what they are, why I use them in my practice, how they work in the body, and what they can do (based on scientific research) to optimize your quality of life.

What Does "Bioidentical" Mean?

First things first: let's perform some definitional housekeeping before we get into the intricacies of bioidentical hormones.

The term "bioidentical" is a joining of the prefix "bio," meaning "life," and "identical," meaning "matching" (as in "identical twins").

What this means from the perspective of molecular science is that **bioidentical hormones match exactly in structure and function the naturally occurring hormones in the human body**.

Specialized pharmacies compound bioidentical hormones out of plant products (soy and/or wild yams). Unlike synthetic hormones, which are often made using much more—let's put it kindly—*exotic* manufacturing methods, bioidentical hormones are fully natural and, therefore, safer and more effective. (This is not merely my opinion as a hormone expert with decades of experience; as we will see, mountains of scientific evidence, growing by the day, provide the proof.)

The therapeutic process of administering bioidentical hormones to augment natural hormone levels (*my specialty at LowTE Florida*) is called **bioidentical hormone replacement therapy** or simply **BHRT for short**.

BHRT is also sometimes called in the clinical literature "compounded bioidentical hormone therapy," or CBHT.

From here on out, for the sake of brevity, I'll use the acronym BHRT to refer to the work we do at LowTE Florida.

The Bioidentical Hormone Breakthrough

Synthetic hormones—pharmaceutical formulations creating artificial, or synthetic, analogs that roughly resemble human hormones—got their start in medicine back in the early 20th century and were widely used throughout the last hundred years (including in the flawed 2002 Women's Health Initiative study we debunked earlier).

Bioidentical hormones, in addition to being safer and more effective, are also newer in the Western medical and public consciousness, despite being first identified and extracted for therapy in the 1930s by a Canadian researcher named James Collip. Aggressive pharmaceutical marketing campaigns, run by well-funded corporations that dominated the relatively young pharmaceutical industry at the time, which promoted synthetic hormones more conducive to mass-production at scale like Premarin®, overshadowed and sidelined bioidentical hormones, despite their greater track record of efficacy and safety.

As a result, to this day, many mainstream medical institutions have still not adopted the use of bioidentical hormones. But the good news is too good to keep hidden forever; as the evidence becomes undeniable and the benefits, they offer over synthetic hormones are made clear, even the most stubborn medical institutions and providers will adopt their use in good time.

The documented risks associated with estrogen therapy for menopausal women have overwhelmingly related to synthetic estrogen, often made using pregnant horse urine (Premarin®) or pregnant horse urine and synthetic progesterone called progestin (Prempro® and Premphase®). On the other hand, specialized compounders derive bioidentical hormones from plant sources (Mexican yams and soy).

Now, let's put our molecular biologist hats on briefly as we get specific in terms of what makes bioidentical hormones so efficacious and desirable over their synthetic competitors.

What Makes Bioidentical Hormones Superior to Synthetic Hormones?

I mentioned previously that the defining feature, and major advantage, of bioidentical hormones is their *exact* molecular matchup with the hormones naturally found in the body.

Your body literally doesn't know the difference between *exogenous* (meaning sourced from outside the body) bioidentical hormones and *endogenous* (meaning sourced from inside the body) hormones. It's all the same to your tissues, organs, and cells, and it's all nourishing IF they are bioidentical.

This means that, by definition, due to how the body processes and reacts to bioidentical hormones introduced through therapy, **they work more effectively while producing fewer and milder side effects** than synthetic alternatives.

Interest in bioidentical hormones, as I mentioned earlier, spiked following the flawed 2002 Women's Health Initiative study that we discussed in the prior chapter (one that purported to demonstrate risks associated with HRT for menopausal women, but which was later debunked due to errors in the study design).

We don't need to rehash the details of the study (feel free to return to the last chapter to find out why it was, in fact, flawed). The point here is that, because the researchers in the WHI study used synthetic hormones given orally, one of the net impacts to the field of hormone therapy over the ensuing years was that bioidentical hormones gained popularity as women looked elsewhere, beyond conventional pharmaceuticals, for answers. They gave the wrong hormones (synthetic), wrong dose (not personalized), and the wrong delivery system (oral). Bioidentical hormone pellets are the safest way to get hormones into your body!

The emphasis here regarding bioidentical hormones should be on the term *natural*, for the reasons explained above as well as the reasons we'll explore in the upcoming section in terms of bioidentical hormones vs. steroids.

Regarding the aforementioned 2002 Women's Health Initiative study, the overbroad conclusions of which have since been recanted, a wealth of scientific evidence points the accusatory finger for the poor results in large part at progestin synthetic form of the female sex hormone progesterone. Progestin (and synthetic estrogen) is responsible for the adverse events that the researchers of that study noted.

Mainstream medical practitioners (many of whom prescribed unnatural hormone drugs for decades) and the FDA (which still allows these dangerous unnatural hormones to be sold) are now at the forefront urging aging women to avoid their prolonged use.

In fact, not only does the data show that, unlike risky synthetic hormones, bioidentical hormones do *not* raise cancer risk. The research demonstrates they actually *lower* cancer risk. We return once again to the Life Extension Magazine whitepaper:

> *"Numerous studies have demonstrated an increased risk of breast cancer with the use of non-bioidentical progestins. However, the use of bioidentical progesterone has not been associated with an increased risk of breast cancer. Quite the contrary, research has revealed that bioidentical progesterone decreases the risk of breast cancer.* ***In a study published in the journal Breast Cancer Research and Treatment, 80,000 postmenopausal women using various forms of HRT were followed for more than 8 years. Women who used estrogen in combination with non-bioidentical progestins had a 69% increased risk of breast cancer, compared to women who had never used HRT. However, for women who used bioidentical progesterone in combination with estrogen, the increased risk of breast cancer was completely eliminated with a***

> ***significant reduction in breast cancer risk compared with non-bioidentical progestin use.*** *"*

It is for the above reasons, as well as others I have already described in prior sections of this book and more to come, that I only prescribe bioidentical hormones estrogen (estradiol), testosterone, and progesterone in my clinical work.

Hormone therapy, like all forms of medicine, is only as good as the ingredients and protocols it employs. There are no shortcuts in the delivery of high-quality anti-aging medicine, and I take none with my patients.

Overlooked by mainstream medicine is a plethora of research findings indicating that women may more safely benefit from individualized doses of natural estrogens and progesterone over their lifetime*. Almost completely ignored are lifestyle changes (such as assuring optimal vitamin D status and cruciferous vegetable intake) that may prevent and even reverse the kind of damage to cell regulatory genes inflicted by some estrogenic compounds.*

In its exposition on the raging information war both within the industry and in public-facing media related to bioidentical vs. synthetic hormones, "The Unscientific Bioidentical Hormone Debate," Life Extension Magazine [4] elaborates further on the harmful impacts of synthetic hormones, citing the lack of enzymes found in the human body to safely break down and process horse estrogens (the foundation of synthetic estrogen):

> *"Most appalling are the innuendos that bioidentical hormones are no different than FDA-approved Premarin® and Prempro®. Both Premarin® and Prempro® contain horse estrogen extracted from pregnant mares' urine.* ***Unlike bioidentical estrogen creams that provide the hormones found naturally in the human female body, horse estrogen contains equilin and other equine estrogens found exclusively in horses****.*

> ***The human female body contains enzymes to metabolize the natural proportion of estriol, estradiol, and estrone, but not horse estrogens such as equilin.*** *These horse estrogens produce estrogenic effects that are much more potent and longer lasting than those produced by natural human estrogens."*

As a layperson, the nitty-gritty mechanics of bioidentical progesterone vs. synthetic progestin notwithstanding, it should be intuitively understood that the body would respond more favorably to therapies using forms of hormones that are fully identical to those that occur naturally in the body rather than synthetic analogs produced using horse estrogens or pharmaceutical chemicals.

Bioidentical Hormones and Synthetic Steroids: What's the Difference and Why Does It Matter?

Because testosterone has the potential to dramatically improve physical performance in terms of stamina, muscle mass, and strength, illegal steroid use is common in the United States, particularly among athletes looking for a competitive edge.

This is how the United States Drug Enforcement Administration (DEA)the law enforcement body tasked with combatting the illegal trade of steroids defines the term [5]:

> *"Anabolic steroids are synthetically produced variants of the naturally occurring male hormone testosterone that are abused in an attempt to promote muscle growth, enhance athletic or other physical performance, and improve physical appearance.*
>
> *Testosterone, trenbolone, oxymetholone, methandrostenolone, nandrolone, stanozolol, boldenone, and oxandrolone are some of the anabolic steroids that are most commonly encountered by United States law enforcement…*

Steroids are ingested orally, injected intramuscularly, or applied to the skin. ***The doses abused are often 10 to 100 times higher than the approved therapeutic and medical treatment dosages****."*

As the DEA is alluding to here, the name of the anti-aging hormone optimization game is not merely jacking your testosterone levels as high as humanly possible a recipe for severe health effects and possibly even death but, rather, getting them into the optimal range.

Here are the differences between black market steroids and bioidentical hormones:

- Bioidentical hormones are legal when provided by a licensed healthcare provider. Anabolic steroids are illegal to use or sell in the United States, subject to enforcement by federal and state and local police agencies
- Bioidentical hormones are natural, with a proven track record of safety. Illegal steroids are synthetic, highly dangerous, and associated with numerous negative health effects, including potentially fatal cardiovascular (heart) events like heart attack or stroke, infertility, sexual dysfunction (impotence), and psychiatric disturbances
- The dosing (which is critical for success) of legal bioidentical hormones is monitored and regulated by a licensed healthcare provider like me in my clinical practice at LowTE Florida. Illegal steroids dosing is left up to guesswork, often, again, involving the use of dangerously high levels of the drug

For the sake of your health and freedom, I beg of you to *never* attempt to regulate your hormones on your own without the appropriate diagnostic and routine blood-monitoring care required. If you have a testosterone deficiency and can benefit from BHRT, we can work together to get your levels right in a safe and effective manner, without incurring the consequences of off-the-charts fluctuations in T counts that result so often in heart attacks, infertility, and the other negative health effects described above.

My goal with hormone therapy has always been to give *the right hormones (bioidentical), the right dose (personalized), and the right delivery system (pellets).*

Hormone optimization is an exact science that requires a team of skilled, experienced, and well-researched hormone experts like the one we have assembled at LowTE Florida to optimize hormones safely.

Getting Down to Brass Tacks

With the introduction to bioidentical hormones out of the way, in the upcoming chapter, we'll get down to the health benefits and breakthroughs that my patients and millions of others around the world have reaped through the careful administration of BHRT.

We'll survey the proven benefits of bioidentical hormones for each of the sexes and you'll hear personal accounts of health transformation in mind, body, and spirit from real-life patients whom I've had the privilege of serving in my LowTE Florida office and who, as a result of our work together, have turned their anti-aging dreams into a healthy-aging reality.

References

[1] McCullough, M. (1998). Hormone Options. Chicago Tribune.

[2] Flies, J., Ko, M., et al. (2011). Bioidentical Hormone Therapy. Mayo Clinic Proceedings. https://www.ncbi.nlm.nih.gov/pmc/articles/PMC3127562/

[3] Life Extension Magazine. (2009). Bioidentical Hormones. Life Extension Magazine. https://www.lifeextension.com/magazine/2009/10/bioidentical-hormones

[4] Faloon, William. (2009). The Unscientific Bioidentical Hormone Debate. Life Extension Magazine. https://www.lifeextension.com/magazine/2009/10/the-unscientific-bioidentical-hormone-debate

[5] Drug Enforcement Administration. (n.d.) Steroids. https://www.dea.gov/factsheets/steroids

Chapter VI
Bioidentical Hormone Therapy for Women

Traditional medicine has not been nice to the aging woman. When discussing your symptoms of declining hormones, you may hear something like "this is normal aging just get used to it," which means you will be aging like an old apple you left on the counter 3 months ago! That is not how I want to age! Or they may prescribe you a synthetic hormone replacement with the thought of giving you the smallest dose for the shortest amount of time. Great. After 50 you get to feel good for a minute then they will take it away from you! Or, even worse, they may prescribe you an antidepressant! You weren't depressed you have hot flashes from the declining estrogen in your body! Why not treat the root of the problem? You may have another 50+ years to live, don't you want them to be fabulous? I do!

For the average woman reading this in her sixties, fifties, forties, or even thirties, you likely don't need me to expound on the widespread prevalence of menopause or its negative effects on women's quality of life.

You've most likely experienced them firsthand.

So, I'll make this crash course on menopause short and sweet. Here are some key facts on menopause:

- Approximately 1.3 million American women will develop the symptoms of menopause in any given year
- **As of 2025**, as the global population advances in age, up to **1.2 billion women worldwide will be in menopause**
- The average age of onset for menopause is 51 years. Some women develop it earlier and some later
- As many as 5% of women enter menopause before the age of 40. This is termed "early menopause"

- Given the average lifespan, a woman will statistically be in menopause for about 40% of her life
- Certain health conditions and procedures, such as the surgical removal of the ovaries called in clinical settings an "oophorectomy" may trigger early menopause

From a clinical perspective, for the diagnosis of "menopause" to be made, a woman must have gone 12 months without a period. At Low TE Florida, we can confirm or make the diagnosis evaluating certain lab values.

However, many women, before entering menopause, experience irregular periods, sometimes with months-long gaps between each one. This is called "perimenopause" and may last months or even years before progressing into menopause.

"Post menopause" refers to the stage following menopause, after a woman has not had her period for more than 12 months.

To summarize, the three stages of menopause are:

- Perimenopause
- Menopause
- Post menopause

The symptoms of perimenopause, menopause, and post menopause can be wide-ranging (remembering that estrogen receptors are found in every organ and tissue). These can be physical, mental, and emotional. They include but are not limited to:

- Hot flashes
- Night sweats
- Irregular periods
- Diminished sex drive (libido)
- Painful intercourse
- Loss of bladder control (incontinence)
- Sleep problems (insomnia)
- Cognitive challenges (aka "brain fog")
- Memory issues

- Mood swings
- Depression
- Anxiety

Sometimes, because the symptoms associated with menopause can be general (non-specific), your doctor might mistake them as associated with another condition aside from menopause. This is, once again, why it's critical to seek out the care of an experienced hormone expert (healthcare provider who specializes in hormones) for an accurate diagnosis and resolution.

The primary precipitating cause of menopause is the lack of eggs for the ovaries to release (unlike male sperm, which are regularly produced in large numbers, female eggs are finite).

As a result of the lack of eggs, the menstrual cycle (period) stops. Estrogen levels drop, which has the downstream effect of spiking follicle-stimulating hormone (FSH) and luteinizing hormone (LH) and causing other hormonal disruptions, which can cause severe and debilitating symptoms. (As I explained in a prior chapter, the body's 50+ hormones exist in a complex and delicate balance. So, when estrogen is removed, the broader impacts on the hormone system can be wide-ranging.)

Aside from age-related declines in fertility, menopause can also be triggered by:

- Certain cancer treatments like radiation therapy and chemotherapy
- Ovarian insufficiency (poor ovarian function)
- Oophorectomy (the surgical removal of the ovaries)

All that said, menopause isn't just a health issue although it is primarily that. It's also a major social and economic issue, one that harms women's ability to earn an income and advance their careers!

As an example of what I'm talking about, a comprehensive study published last year in the Mayo Clinic Proceedings [1] found that working American women lose out on no less than $1.8 billion in lost wages due to menopause-related work stoppages each year:

"Women are a vital part of the global workforce and economy. This study identified an association between menopause symptoms and adverse work outcomes, including lost work productivity. The severity of menopause symptoms strongly predicted the odds of an adverse work outcome. Based on this analysis, ***the estimated annual cost associated with lost days of work related to menopause symptoms among US women aged 45 to 60 years is $1.8 billion****...*

The findings of this study highlight a critical need to improve the medical treatment provided to women with menopause symptoms."

Despite how common and debilitating menopause is, shocking numbers of women never seek out treatment for their condition, nor are they educated sufficiently on their options for treatment, even though therapy with bioidentical hormones of the kind I offer at LowTE Florida is proven to work for nearly all women experiencing the symptoms of menopause.

Consider these shocking figures by way of Forbes [2]:

"The State of Menopause Study, conducted with 1,039 women ages 40 to 65 across the United States, showed that nearly ***one-third (29%) of women never sought information about menopause*** *before they experienced it.*

Nearly half (45%) the women surveyed didn't know the difference between perimenopause—the transitional period leading up to menopause—and menopause *itself, the biological process that marks the end of a woman's menstrual cycles.*

One-fifth (20%) of women surveyed had experienced symptoms for a year or more before being assessed by a healthcare provider *and 34% had never been formally assessed or diagnosed as menopausal.*

> ***Most (73%) women reported that they were not currently treating their menopause****, which included hot flashes (16%), weight gain (15%), difficulties with sleep (14%), and night sweats (14%), among others."*

I consider these shocking statistics a reflection of the tragic failure of the healthcare system to educate and empower women regarding the most common chronic health condition of all, which will affect virtually all women at some point in their lives.

Much of the cause for this lack of awareness and proper treatment of menopause, I would argue, can be chalked up to the long-standing social stigma around the condition, despite its universal prevalence among the female population, as explained via The Lancet [3]:

> ***"Stigma, embarrassment, a lack of public awareness, and miscommunication mean that for many women, menopause is either borne in quiet suffering or else over-medicalized*** *as nothing more than a hormone deficiency requiring estrogen replacement. Menopause is a natural part of ageing that affects 50% of the population. Yet, this fact is not reflected in many societies, and their health systems. The long-standing neglect of menopause and silence around it must change."*

Let's break through the wall of silence together and end the stigma and lack of education surrounding menopause once and for all. There is no justification for menopause-induced shame nor is there any legitimate reason that it should go untreated in the 21st century.

The over-arching message I aim to deliver with this book, as I introduce my readers and future patients to the miracle of bioidentical hormone replacement therapy, is this: **there is no law that says you must suffer this way** not now, , not with the advanced and inexpensive diagnostic and therapeutic tools we have at hand.

Given how safe, effective, accessible, and increasingly affordable hormone therapy is, there is no moral justification for 73% of women experiencing menopause to not reap the benefits of bioidentical hormones and get their lives back.

Life is too short to feel like *&#%! I believe you want whatever time you have left on earth to be fabulous!! You deserve a great life!

The Proven Benefits of Bioidentical Estradiol (Estrogen) For Women

Here's what none other than Oprah Winfrey herself had to say about what bioidentical estrogen did for her mental and physical health, via U.S. News and World Report [4]:

> *"A January [2009] Oprah show featured both discussing their positive experiences on the hormones, which came across as a virtual cure-all for aging. [Bestselling author Suzanne] Somers, who takes much higher doses of bioidentical hormones than most experts recommend, believes that the supplements keep her young and feeling sexy and are preventing her breast cancer from coming back. On her website,* ***Winfrey writes, "After one day on bioidentical estrogen, I felt the veil lift. After three days, the sky was bluer, my brain was no longer fuzzy, my memory was sharper. I was literally singing and had a skip in my step."***

The most effective form of bioidentical estrogen, which I utilize exclusively for my patients receiving therapy at my LowTE Florida clinic, **is bioidentical estradiol**.

Taking each unique benefit of bioidentical hormone replacement therapy (BHRT) with bioidentical estrogen in the form of estradiol one at a time, let's survey, based on publicly available clinical data, the health transformations that these potent compounds afford women experiencing menopause.

Bioidentical Estrogen Improves Sleep Quality in Women

Impaired sleep (the inability to fall asleep and/or stay asleep throughout the night) is one of the more common symptoms of menopause.

And, because lack of proper sleep has reverberating mental and physical health impacts across multiple domains, it's a huge issue that must be remedied, which I do for my female patients at my LowTE Florida office. If you don't have a good night's sleep it is impossible to have a great day.

BHRT with bioidentical estrogen is proven to improve sleep quality in menopausal women, as demonstrated in the following 7-month study published in the American Journal of Obstetrics and Gynecology [5]:

> *"**Estrogen replacement therapy improved sleep quality, facilitated falling asleep, and decreased nocturnal restlessness and awakenings.** The subjects were **less tired in the mornings and in the daytime** when taking estrogen replacement therapy. **Estrogen-induced sleep improvement was associated with alleviation of vasomotor symptoms,** alleviation of somatic symptoms, **and alleviation of mood symptoms** on estrogen replacement therapy."*

Good-quality sleep is a pillar of any effective anti-aging strategy, critical for optimal mental and physical health. My LowTE Florida female patients receiving bioidentical estrogen therapy reap the numerous benefits of improved sleep.

Bioidentical Estrogen Strengthens Bones and Prevents Osteoporosis in Women

As we age, the risk of bone fractures increases, as does the likelihood that broken bones will lead to long-term disability. Indeed, a fractured hip late in life could potentially prove fatal.

Therefore, strengthening bones to prevent osteoporosis (the clinical term for age-related bone weakening) is an anti-aging non-negotiable. And we achieve just that for my menopausal patients at LowTE Florida.

Lack of estrogen, research shows, is the primary driver of osteoporosis in older women. Conversely, estrogen therapy is the number one therapy to reverse the condition and restore bone density to optimal levels.

Let's take a look at the following report from Menopause Review [6]:

> *"**Postmenopausal osteoporosis and related fractures** are a serious health threat... and about **half of elderly women will have long-term disability, morbidity and death after a fracture...***
>
> *Despite **decades of accumulated evidence demonstrating that HRT is the most effective therapy for the prevention of osteoporosis and related fractures,** the United States' Food and Drug Administration (FDA) and the European Medicine Evaluation Agency (EMEA), have recommended not to use HRT as the first-line therapy for prevention of osteoporosis. This advice was based mainly on the presentation and interpretation of **the [Women's Health Initiative] data that were greatly revised by the menopause community*...**"*

(This excerpt is in reference to the deeply flawed and later-revised 2002 Women's Health Initiative study that we debunked in an earlier chapter in this book, "The Forgotten Healing Art of Hormone Replacement Therapy.")

Continuing with Menopause Review:

> *"Years ago, **we forecasted that the drop in HRT use could have caused an increase in fragility fractures in elderly women**. In a recent study, Karim et al. have measured the impact of HRT cessation on the incidence of hip fracture in a large longitudinal study including 80 955 postmenopausal women. In this huge cohort of postmenopausal women followed for 6.5 years, **HRT discontinuation was associated with a 55% increase in the risk of hip fracture alone**."*

And so we see here the real-world consequences, using hard data, of flawed science of the kind found in the 2002 WHI study, which resulted in millions of women foregoing life-enhancing and even life-saving hormone therapy, in turn leading to a 55% increase in the rates of hip fractures a form of trauma that, again, for many older women, is a literal death sentence.

More from Menopause Review:

> *"The use **of HRT for osteoporosis prevention is based on biology, epidemiology, animal and preclinical data, observational studies and randomized, clinical trials,** and thus **bone protection has been included among the benefits of HRT** in recent recommendations. In fact, **osteoporosis prevention can actually be considered as a major additional effect in perimenopausal women who use HRT** for treatment of climacteric symptoms"*

As with all the documented benefits of BHRT with bioidentical estrogen, none of this is guesswork.

Clinical tests such as dual-energy X-ray absorptiometry (DXA) graphically depict bone density, and we consistently see superior bone density in female patients who receive hormone therapy at LowTE Florida vs. those who don't.

One patient comes to mind. She was crying on the phone with me after her bone scan. She had been on BHRT pellets with me for several years. She was crying with joy her numbers were improving on her scan. She was afraid she was going to have a horrible old age like her mother who suffered with osteoporosis. Besides estradiol, we have learned that testosterone actually re-lays bone helping us to have healthy bones as we age so the combination of testosterone and estradiol is just what your bones need to be healthy. It's one thing for me to read about this in the literature, but to see improved bone scans time and time again after initiating BHRT is something else.

Bioidentical Estrogen Improves Cardiovascular Health and Prevents Heart Disease in Women

Cardiovascular disease (also referred to as CVD or heart disease) is the reigning number one killer of women (as well as men) worldwide and has been for decades.

Modern medicine, as I have pointed out before, is great at achieving certain healthcare wins, like treating acute infections or repairing broken bones.

However, modern medicine, unfortunately, has *not* proven itself capable of preventing or reversing chronic illness, and that includes heart disease.

A large part of the solution to age-related heart disease is hormones, including estrogen, which play an important role in maintaining heart health in women. Without enough estrogen to nourish the heart, as happens during menopause, women are at increased risk of developing heart disease.

Let's briefly survey research published in Current Opinion in Nephrology and Hypertension [7]:

> ***"Cardiovascular disease (CVD) is the leading cause of death in the United States*** *and differs significantly depending on age and sex. Observational studies have demonstrated that* ***both the incidence of CVD and resultant morbidity and mortality are much less in premenopausal women*** *compared to age-matched men, and* ***this sex advantage for women becomes far less or disappears with increased age and reduced estrogen levels after menopause.*** *Observational studies also show that* ***postmenopausal women who receive hormone replacement therapy (HRT) have a lower rate of CVD and cardiac death than those not receiving HRT."***

The heart health-optimizing effects of BHRT are not guesswork; we can measure the effectiveness of BHRT with bioidentical estrogen for stabilizing and optimizing heart health with several metrics, including blood pressure, c-reactive protein levels, and cholesterol levels, all of which are consistently improved in menopausal women following therapy.

Research published in the American Heart Journal [8], for instance, demonstrates clinically significant reductions in blood pressure in postmenopausal women receiving estrogen infusions:

> ***"Coronary heart disease (CHD) in women is strongly associated with estrogen deprivation.*** *For example, risk for CHD increases dramatically after menopause...*
>
> *Postmenopausal women on long-term HRT were recruited along with a control group of postmenopausal women not on HRT. These women were divided into higher versus lower risk for CHD on the basis of resting [blood pressure]...*
>
> ***HRT eliminates the cumulative effect of resting [blood pressure]*** *and family history on BP reactivity, suggesting that* ***the circulatory effects of estrogen replacement may operate,*** *at least in part,* ***through normalization of BP reactivity in higher-risk postmenopausal women."***

In more basic terms, in postmenopausal women with high resting blood pressure, hormone therapy improves circulation and reduces blood pressure, which I consistently see firsthand in my clinical practice at LowTE Florida.

On the cholesterol front, bioidentical estrogen therapy likewise delivers massive benefits for menopausal women by lowering LDL cholesterol levels (the "bad" form of cholesterol associated with heart attacks and stroke), via the American Journal of Medicine [9]:

> *"Continuous combined* ***hormone-replacement therapy can produce significant and therapeutic reductions in LDL cholesterol levels in hypercholesterolemic postmenopausal women.*** *After internists become familiar with the expected side effects and their time course, this regimen may provide* ***an effective approach in the management of hypercholesterolemia in postmenopausal women*** *who have not undergone hysterectomy."*

("Hypercholesterolemia" is the clinical term for "high cholesterol.")

Bioidentical Estrogen Improves Exercise Capacity and Athletic Performance in Women

Staying active late in life is essential for longevity and maintaining a high quality of life.

But it's not always easy or enjoyable to exercise during or after menopause because the drop in sex hormones results in impaired athletic performance/exercise capacity.

BHRT with bioidentical estrogen is proven to restore women's physical prowess, motivating treated individuals to hit the gym, the trail, or the slopes however you get your kicks, so to speak.

In the following study published, once again, in our trusted resource, the American Heart Journal [10]researchers studied the impact of estrogen therapy on 248 postmenopausal women with an average age of 63 years.

The team controlled for what scientists call "confounding" variables such as "physical activity level, body mass index, waist-to-hip ratio, presence of osteoporosis, and family history of heart disease" meaning they factored these metrics into their analysis so that they were **measuring only the direct effect of estrogen therapy on physical performance** *(apologies for the brief clinical research lesson, but I love teaching my patients how to critically read literature to empower themselves to consume and apply all of the scientific knowledge out there).*

This is what the researchers found:

> ***"We measured maximal oxygen uptake* (MVO (2)) and anaerobic threshold*** *as objective markers of exercise capacity...* ***We found that fitness,*** *as measured by MVO (2) and anaerobic threshold,* ***was significantly greater in women who had used HRT currently or in the past compared with women who had never used HRT.*** *This difference in fitness was not confounded by age or physical activity level...*

> ***Estrogen replacement therapy is associated with increased exercise capacity as measured by MVO (2) and anaerobic threshold****... This finding is consistent with the beneficial effect of short-term estrogen administration on improved endothelium-dependent and endothelium-independent vasodilation."*

*Maximal oxygen uptake, sometimes called "VO2 max," is one of the tops, if not the most important, markers of physical acumen and overall cardiovascular (heart) capacity for handling exercise-related stress.

Accordingly, these findings are profound in their implications regarding BHRT with bioidentical estrogen's beneficial impacts on women's athletic performance.

Applying theory to practice, the menopausal and postmenopausal women who visit my LowTE Florida office for BHRT with bioidentical estrogen, without fail, report enhanced stamina and strength as well as greater vitality and enthusiasm to remain active, no matter what their chronological age might be.

Triathlons in your sixties, seventies, or eighties? No problem!

Bioidentical Estrogen Improves Mental Health and Fights Depression and Anxiety in Women

Mental health drags are among the most pervasive and debilitating downstream effects of menopause, which often encompass a cornucopia of related symptoms: mood swings, depression, anxiety, loss of interest in activities you used to love, etc.

In a review of the deleterious effects of menopause on cognition and mental health, published in 2022 in Best Practice & Research Clinical Obstetrics & Gynecology [11], the researchers noted:

> ***"Cognitive and mood changes are frequently mentioned as complaints before, during and after menopausal transition.*** *There is substantial biological evidence for such associations to occur, as there are many mechanisms through which* ***estrogens can affect***

> ***the brain:*** *by regulating metabolism, increasing cerebral blood flow and dendritic outgrowth, by acting on nerve growth factors through the co-localization of receptors via neurotransmitter synthesis and turnover and many more…* ***Hormone treatment (HT) including estrogens could potentially reverse these psychological issues."***

From a basic biological perspective, these cognitive and emotional changes are to be expected, since the brain is chock-full of estrogen receptors that go undernourished once circulating estrogen levels dry up during menopause.

It naturally follows, then, that replenishing circulating estrogen to the brain would result in improved cognition and mental health, which is what we see in the clinical literature as well as what I see on a personal, practical level in my LowTE Florida clinic.

For instance, here is a commentary about estrogen therapy for mental health symptoms associated with menopause from The Journal of Affective Disorders [12]:

> ***"Clinical studies indicate that estrogen replacement improves mood and increases the sense of well-being in post-menopausal*** *women with no or mild depressive symptoms...* ***Interestingly, estrogen can remedy the symptoms of perimenopausal depression*** *providing support for the idea that ovarian hormones are involved in the expression of the disorder. Recently, Schmidt et al. (2000)* ***demonstrated the beneficial effects of estrogen replacement in perimenopausal depression to be independent of its ability to reduce the sleep disturbances and the distress of hot flushes."***

My female LowTE Florida patients many of whom have tried and met no success with conventional treatments for depression like SSRI antidepressants consistently benefit from remarkable mental health rebounds following BHRT with bioidentical estrogen, which typically become manifest after a month or so of therapy. Many of my patients have been able to wean themselves off their medications for anxiety and depression once their hormones are optimized.

Bioidentical Estrogen Optimizes Cognition and Memory in Women

Dovetailing with lifted depression, improved mood, and reduced anxiety levels, menopausal women receiving BHRT with bioidentical estrogen also benefit from improved cognition and memory.

The authors of the following 2021 study published in Human Brain Mapping [13] recruited 524 women between the ages of 71-94 years old and studied the effects of estrogen therapy on gray and white matter as measured by brain scans:

> *"The main finding of this paper is that* ***a history of estrogen use*** *in a large cohort of* ***elderly women was associated with larger gray and white matter volumes, in brain regions relevant to cognitive function*** *including frontal, temporal, and parietal lobes.* ***These findings remained statistically significant regardless of time point of estrogen use history, cardiovascular risk factors, genetic make-up or lifestyle factors*** *previously studied such as physical activity…*
>
> *These findings are from a relatively large group of women, compared with most prior studies demonstrating a relationship between estrogen and brain structure.*
>
> ***Similar to our results, a study of 40 healthy postmenopausal women****—of whom 17 were either using or had a history of estrogen use—****showed greater gray matter volumes on structural MRI*** *of the frontal, temporal, and parietal lobes including the hippocampus with voxel-based morphometry."*

Greater gray matter volumes are an excellent indicator of better cognitive health, as brain shrinkage is closely tied to cognitive decline.

Bioidentical Estrogen Minimizes Risk of Dementia and Other Neurological Diseases in Women

Finally, closing out the mental and cognitive benefits of BHRT with bioidentical estrogen for menopausal women, let's take a look at the protective effects it exerts in terms of preventing cognitive decline and associated illnesses.

Most of us personally know a loved one who has battled cognitive decline late in life, whether in the form of Alzheimer's disease or other forms of dementia.

However, the biological reality is that the table for cognitive decline is set decades before the symptoms become noticeable, much less debilitating.

The key, therefore, to improving health outcomes in this domain is to catch and prevent the decline as early as possible; "an ounce of prevention is worth a pound of cure," as the saying goes.

Returning once more to the Human Brain Mapping study:

> *"Declining estrogen levels for women in all stages of menopause can affect memory and risk of Alzheimer's Disease (AD), emphasizing a role for hormone therapy (HT)…*
>
> *Alzheimer's disease (AD) is the most common neurodegenerative cause of dementia;* ***female sex is a key risk factor for AD, particularly after menopause and precipitous declines in estrogen levels…***
>
> ***Memory is influenced by the relative expression of estrogen receptors as they interact with estradiol.*** *Given the postmenopausal decline in levels of estradiol and potentially beneficial hormones such as progesterone, one hypothesis is that boosting these levels through HT may reduce AD risk in women…*

Long-term postmenopausal HT was associated with a lower risk of any dementia diagnosis including AD."

So, if you're a woman interested in optimizing and protecting your brain health late into life and who isn't? And staving off neurodegenerative conditions like Alzheimer's disease, there is no single superior therapeutic intervention than BHRT with bioidentical estrogen in tandem with regular exercise, a clean diet, and clean sleep habits.

I have one patient that says she needs her pellet therapy to help reduce her chances of developing Alzheimer's Disease. She says she can't afford to get Alzheimer's because she is taking care of both of her parents that are suffering from Alzheimer's Disease. Wow. She did the research.

Bioidentical Estrogen Decreases Risk of Tooth Decay and Tooth Loss in Women

We all want a set of pearly whites and it's only natural, as healthy teeth are a sign of overall health and therefore are a powerful, universal indicator of attractiveness.

Good dental health isn't just an aesthetic concern in terms of keeping a bright, white smile; you might be surprised to learn poor dental hygiene is also implicated in numerous long-term chronic illnesses like heart disease.

Furthermore, you might not immediately think of dental health in relation to menopause, but, in fact, lower estrogen and all its downstream effects can wreak havoc in this regard.

Let's have a look-see at the following research published in the Annals of Medical and Health Sciences Research [14]:

> ***"Oral discomfort is found in many menopausal women*** *in addition to general climacteric complaints. The principal pre- and post-menopausal oral symptoms are dry mouth, sensation of painful mouth (PM) due to various causes and less frequently burning mouth syndrome (BMS)...*

It is very important for all patients moving towards the age of menopause or currently experiencing this change to understand how menopause could affect their oral health and what can be done to avoid related complications like periodontal disease and tooth decay...

In post-menopausal women, alterations of the oral cavity are related to the hormone alterations *that characterize these patients and to physiological aging of the oral tissues,* ***potentially giving rise to periodontitis****, BMS and xerostomia."*

"HT is extensively used to alleviate menopause related oral symptoms for the well-being of the women treated," the researchers add.

Here we have a study examining the relationship between estrogen therapy and tooth loss/denture use in nearly 4,000 menopausal women, published via Archives of Internal Medicine [15]:

"The recognized benefit of estrogen replacement therapy (ERT) in postmenopausal osteoporosis prompted review of the Leisure World Cohort Study regarding ***the effects of [estrogen replacement therapy] on tooth loss and the need for dentures*** *in older women...*

After adjusting for age, ***tooth loss and rates of edentia were significantly lower in estrogen users*** *than in nonusers. The proportion of women with edentia decreased with increasing duration of ERT.* ***Denture wearing was also less common in estrogen users*** *than in nonusers and decreased with increasing duration of ERT."*

("Edentia" is a clinical term that means "lack of teeth.")

What could be better, from a dental health perspective, than keeping your own natural, healthy teeth deep into your golden years? If, as a woman, that sounds good to you, then sufficient estrogen with the aid of bioidentical hormone replacement therapy is an essential prerequisite.

The bottom line is that standard hygiene practices such as regular flossing, brushing, avoiding excessive sugar intake, etc.in combination with BHRT with bioidentical estrogen of the kind that my female patients at LowTE Florida receive is the best strategy for women experiencing menopause to maintain a healthy set of teeth late into life.

Bioidentical Estrogen Improves Metabolism and Lowers Diabetes Risk in Women

Metabolism, as we discussed in a previous chapter, is the process by which the body processes, uses, and stores energy.

Fast, efficient metabolism (the kind of metabolism you want) means that your body effectively turns food into high amounts of energy and doesn't store it as excess body fat. Slow metabolism, on the other hand, means that your body doesn't maintain high energy levels and tends to store calories from food as body fat.

Unfortunately, as women age, our metabolism tends to slow down, resulting in unwanted weight gain. There are numerous reasons for this, but hormones are the biggest of them.

For more on the link between estrogen and metabolism, let's defer to the experts at the University of Chicago Medicine [16]:

> ***"You're eating and exercising as you always have, yet you find yourself gaining weight,*** *especially around your midsection.*
>
> *What's going on?*
>
> *For women in their 40s or 50s,* ***that's likely a sign their body is transitioning to menopause.***
>
> *It's common for those entering this natural stage of life to gain weight and belly fat (sometimes called* ***"menopause belly"****)...*
>
> ***The decrease in estrogen and progesterone,*** *along with aging in* ***general, triggers metabolic changes in the body.*** *One change is*

a decrease in muscle mass, ***resulting in fewer calories being burned.*** *If fewer calories are being burned, fat accumulates."*

"Menopause belly"? Yikes!

But, if low estrogen is the trigger, then higher estrogen via BHRT with bioidentical estrogen is the logical solution, one that consistently delivers results that matter to my LowTE Florida patients.

In research published in the medical journal Maturitas [17], investigators gave one group a placebo and another group (called the "substituted group") estrogen and progesterone, then measured their body weight, waist-to-hip ratio (a major indicator of attractiveness), lipid oxidation (AKA fat burning), cholesterol levels, and other indicators of metabolic health after a period of three months.

Here are the results:

"Total body weight was unaltered after 3 months in the control group, whereas ***a fat-loss of 2.1+/-0.2 kg and a decrease of the waist: hip ratio was observed in the substituted group.*** *In the latter group,* ***a significant increase in lipid oxidation was observed*** *(0.58+/-0.06 mg/kg/min before and 0.75+/-0.04 mg/kg/min after substitution P<0.05),* ***whilst total energy expenditure and thermogenesis were also increased.*** *Glucose, lipid and protein oxidation remained stable during three months in the control group.* ***The insulin response to an oral glucose load diminished by 30% with hormone replacement therapy*** *(102.3+/-32.8 mmicro/l versus 71.4+/-20.0 mmicro/l).* ***Total and LDL-cholesterol improved after hormone replacement therapy*** *whereas plasma triglycerides were not altered.*

Combined hormone replacement therapy not only prevented weight-gain but favored weight-loss by significantly increasing lipid oxidation after 3 months of treatment. It also favorably influenced the insulin response, plasma lipids and energy expenditure."

To recap, bioidentical estrogen therapy may:

- Induces clinically significant weight loss
- Improves hip-to-waist ratio
- Increases fat burning
- Increases energy levels
- Reduces insulin response (important for preventing diabetes and other forms of metabolic dysfunction)
- Reduces harmful cholesterol levels

Again, I ask the rhetorical question: what one drug out there can achieve all these weight loss, cholesterol-lowering, and metabolism-boosting benefits aside from bioidentical estrogen via BHRT?

The answer, of course, is none.

When you're ready to get serious about losing weight, feeling more energetic, and improving your physique, my doors at LowTE Florida are always open.

Bioidentical Estrogen Improves Joint Function and Reduces Joint Pain in Women

Whether you're a tennis player or a grandmother who wants to keep up with her grandkids, paying proper attention to preserving your joint health is critical to staying physically active.

Creaky, painful joints often accompany aging, but they are not by any stretch of the imagination inevitable.

Menopause is associated with numerous chronic health conditions that cause deteriorating joints including, for instance, forms of arthritis such as osteoarthritis.

Over recent years, researchers have developed a greater appreciation for the role that estrogen plays in preventing degenerative conditions of the joints. As such, there is a growing recognition within the anti-aging field of the role of estrogen therapy in correcting them, as surveyed below via Arthritis Research & Therapy [18]:

> *"Osteoarthritis (OA) is a very common chronic disease that affects all joint tissues, causing progressive irreversible damage and, finally, the failure of the joint as an organ...*
>
> ***Among the multiple physio pathological mechanisms*** *involved in OA,* ***those related to sex hormone control have been attracting much attention, in particular*** *those involving* ***estrogens****...*
>
> ***There is increasing evidence that estrogens fulfill a relevant role in maintaining the homeostasis of articular tissues*** *and, hence, of the joint itself...* ***This association indicates a potential protective role for estrogens against the development of OA.****"*

Furthermore, from Frontiers in Physiology [19], estrogen protects joint function in numerous ways, including by maintaining high collagen levels the main connective protein in all connective tissues like ligaments and tendons:

> *"Estrogen has a dramatic effect on musculoskeletal function. Beyond the known relationship between estrogen and bone, it directly affects the structure and function of other musculoskeletal tissues such as muscle, tendon, and ligament. In these other musculoskeletal tissues,* ***estrogen improves muscle mass and strength, and increases the collagen content of connective tissues.****"*

Collagen also helps maintain skin elasticity for a youthful glow, which my patients benefit from following BHRT with bioidentical estrogen.

Like I tell my patients at my LowTE Florida office, depending on the state of your joints, sometimes in the later stages of joint disease expensive and invasive surgeries might be necessary, as in the case of knee replacements, etc.

But as a preventative measure to prevent joint degeneration and maintain healthy joints long after menopause, starting bioidentical estrogen therapy at the first signs of menopause is the most cost-effective, least invasive protective measure any woman can take to protect her joints.

My plea to women over 40 in this regard is: please don't wait for the pain to begin to take care of your joint health when a simple, accessible, inexpensive prophylactic option is on the table, waiting for you to seize it.

Bioidentical Estrogen Improves Libido (Sex Drive) and Sexual Performance for Women

Given that estrogen is the major female sex hormone, it comes as no surprise that estrogen deficiency caused by menopause can have detrimental, potentially severe impacts on women's sexual health.

Some of the common sex-related symptoms of menopause can include, but are not limited to:

- Vaginal dryness
- Vaginal atrophy (atrophic vaginitis), characterized by shrunken, thin, and/or dry vagina
- Painful intercourse
- Loss of libido (loss of interest in sex)

The unique type of bioidentical hormone replacement therapy with bioidentical estrogen that I utilize at my LowTE Florida office is proven to restore sex drive and resolve the above sexual symptoms of menopause.

The causal relationship between menopause and reduced sexual desire/performance in women is well-documented, as explained extensively in the clinical literature for instance, via Hormones and Behavior [20]:

> *"**Menopause-related decrease in sexual desire can be extreme and even debilitating**... Roughly 9-percent of naturally and up to 26-percent of surgically postmenopausal women suffer from a*

> *persistent and distressing lack of sexual desire...* ***Salivary estradiol [is] a significant positive predictor of sexual desire.*** *"*

Moving on to solutions, let's take a look at what BHRT with bioidentical estrogen can do for women's sexual health, by way of the Journal of Women's Health & Gender-Based Medicine [21]:

> *"The availability of different preparations that could replace estrogens and androgens has led to many studies of the use of hormone replacement therapy (HRT) for sexual dysfunction.* ***Dyspareunia* due to vaginal dryness appears to be most responsive to estrogen replacement therapy (ERT)*** *via restoration of vaginal cells, pH, and blood flow."*

*"Dyspareunia" is the medical term for "painful intercourse." Dyspareunia has been described by my patients as painful intercourse that feels like knives or shards of glass in their vaginas. Sexual relations are the glue in relationships. If one partner is unable to have comfortable and enjoyable sex, it will most likely affect the relationship in a bad way. My patients usually say that the dyspareunia is repaired within a few weeks after treatment.

Continuing with the Journal of Women's Health & Gender-Based Medicine:

> *"There also appears to be a significant subgroup of women whose sexual difficulties respond initially to ERT but who subsequently revert to their initial problems, especially when the problem has been loss of libido. For these women,* ***the addition of androgen has proved helpful.*** *"*

Women visiting my LowTE Florida office are often pleasantly surprised to learn that testosterone (androgen) therapy can also be hugely beneficial for the gentler sex, not just for men. We're going to get into this important therapy for women in greater depth later in this chapter.

Bioidentical Estrogen Increases Lifespan and Reduces All-Cause Mortality in Women

Who among us doesn't want to live longer to enjoy retirement, to see our grandkids grow up, or to just soak up all that life has to offer before we move on?

There are many proven ways to increase lifespan including through regular exercise, optimized diet, and healthy sleep habits but, for women experiencing menopause, bioidentical estrogen therapy is among the most effective life-extending strategies.

Let's start off with the negative effects on longevity associated with low estrogen whether due to menopause, surgical removal of the ovaries, or other causes from the JNCI Cancer Spectrum [22]:

> *"Normal healthy aging is characterized by a progressive loss of physiologic function and increased risk of disease and death.* ***Many of the long-term health consequences of normal aging,*** *such as osteoporosis, heart disease, stroke, chronic musculoskeletal complaints, and cognitive impairment,* ***are seen with reduced estrogen environments*** *caused by surgical menopause [or] the natural menopausal transition."*

As the literature from JNCI Cancer Spectrum goes on to explain, estrogen, as the main female sex hormone, regulates and checks the aging process in various ways:

> *"****Estrogen is*** *a* ***key*** *regulator in development and tissue homeostasis across tissues* ***throughout the life span****. Estrogen is* ***involved in*** *regulating mechanisms required for tissue maintenance and repair, such as* ***stem cell division, mitochondrial function, intracellular communication****, and* ***circadian rhythm*****. Alteration and dysregulation of these and other mechanisms are considered hallmarks of the natural aging process."*

*Circadian rhythm is the biological term for "sleep-wake-cycle"; estrogen's integral role in the circadian rhythm is one of the reasons that insomnia is a common symptom in women experiencing menopause.

One study published in the medical journal Menopause [23] examined the life extension benefits of estrogen therapy (ET) in over 8,000 older California women, concluding that "long-term users of ET seem to have a lower death rate in the Leisure World population. The reduction in the risk of death from all causes was 15%. Considering only mortality as the index of therapeutic success or failure, these results suggest that *long-term therapy may extend life.*"

Another study, this one from The Journal of Family Practice [24], likewise studied using an advanced computer model the difference in longevity between postmenopausal women ages 50-65 treated with estrogen as compared to the lifespan of their peers who went without hormone therapy. These are the encouraging results of their inquiry:

> *"Computer simulation by Markov analysis can be applied to current data to estimate the increase in life expectancy obtained from postmenopausal estrogen use and compare them with benefits from other therapies for [coronary artery disease] risk reduction...*
>
> ***Benefits were very favorable when compared with other accepted strategies*** *for [coronary artery disease] risk reduction...*
>
> ***Substantial increases in life expectancy may result from postmenopausal estrogen therapy.*** *These may be* ***equal to or possibly greater than benefits from other well-recognized risk-reduction strategies.****"*

The bottom line on bioidentical estrogen and longevity at this time is this: it is no longer controversial to claim that proper estrogen levels whether naturally occurring or optimized via bioidentical hormone replacement therapy are statistically proven to significantly increase women's lifespan. The verdict is in.

Having established that fact, you might be familiar with the expression "quality over quantity."

My mother recently turned 90 years old. She has had the benefit of hormone replacement throughout her menopausal years (thanks to her daughter!). At 90 she is physically fit, healthy, mentally clear, and thriving. She sings in the choir at church, goes to water aerobics, volunteers at the community theater and has a strong social network. If you drive through her community, you may see her driving her golf cart with her dachshund Elsie at her side. She is proof that hormones throughout the lifetime can give you a good old age. Don't tell her, but I want to be just like her when I grow up!

Of course, our objective in the field of anti-aging medicine that I practice at LowTE Florida is not merely about living *longer*; living *better* is just as important, if not more so.

Coming up, we're going to discuss how bioidentical estrogen via BHRT not only increases menopausal women's lifespan but also enhances its quality so that you can live your best life possible.

Bioidentical Estrogen Improves Quality of Life for Women

The sum of the benefits I have heretofore summarized (in addition to many other beneficial effects that I have omitted for the sake of brevity) is a marked improvement in the quality of life (QoL) index for women receiving BHRT with bioidentical estrogen.

Despite how it might sound, QoL is not merely a subjective, abstract concept; it can be, and is, measured in clinical work using objective metrics.

One study, for instance, published in the British Journal of Obstetrics and Gynecology [25], surveyed over a hundred women experiencing the symptoms of menopause regarding the quality-of-life improvement that they experienced after beginning hormone therapy:

> *"The increase in the quality adjusted life year weight due to hormone replacement therapy for women with mild symptoms was*

0.26 according to the rating scale method and 0.18 according to the time tradeoff method. For women with severe symptoms the quality adjusted life year weight increased by 0.50 according to the rating scale method and by 0.42 according to the time tradeoff method.

***Hormone replacement therapy leads to a major improvement in quality of life for women with menopausal symptoms**... Hormone replacement therapy is economically beneficial for women with menopausal symptoms."*

Similar findings appear in a massive 2020 guideline document for hormone therapy in menopausal women, which reviewed the clinical literature on the subject and was published in the Journal of Menopausal Medicine [26]:

*"Epidemiology research on the QoL and menopause symptoms of women in menopause also showed a similar correlation between the two, but **women receiving [hormone therapy] were shown to have a high QoL** in aspects such as VMS, psychosociological changes, and physical changes. In an evaluation of QoL using the SF-36 questionnaire, **the group receiving [hormone therapy] was shown to have a higher QoL score than the group not receiving [hormone therapy]**. In another study, there was an increase in the score of Women's Health Questionnaire (WHQ) and an improvement of physical symptoms, depression symptoms, and sleep disorder in the treatment group receiving [hormone therapy]."*

I am overjoyed to report the consistent stories of transformed quality of life in my female patients at LowTE Florida following BHRT with bioidentical estrogen. Indeed, hearing these success stories makes all the hard work worthwhile. One patient recently said, "I don't understand why people don't understand that aging with youthful hormone levels is the best thing you can do for yourself for a good old age."

Bioidentical Estrogen and Breast Cancer

Since the Women's Health Initiative study in 2002, it has been a daily struggle educating women on the safety of estrogen. There has been so much misinformation shared that it is a difficult and ongoing task dispelling all the information written that just isn't true. When I first began studying BHRT I asked every expert and hormone professional I met "Is what I am doing causing breast cancer or making cancer grow quicker?" The repeated answer was "absolutely not". The more we learn about estrogen the more we understand how **protective** estrogen (estradiol) is for the breasts! In fact, we have two researchers' production studies showing a 30-40% decreased risk of breast cancer while utilizing our pellet system. I am including a few of the studies in this book.

One thing to keep in mind, I learned during my training that it takes 7-10 years from when the first cell is triggered to develop cancer until you can even diagnose it! ***Also, in five continents, natural bioidentical testosterone has been used to treat breast cancer***. It has been shown to decrease the incidence of breast cancer and shrinks tumors before they are removed. Dr. Rebecca Glaser has published several studies showing how protective our pellet therapy is for the breasts.

We recommend annual mammograms for all our female patients over 40. Not that what we do causes cancer, we just want to know that you are healthy. I have been treating women with estrogen for 30+ years and the percentage of my patients that have had breast cancer is less than women who are not on hormones.

Honestly, out of over 21,000 patients treated I have seen less than 20 breast cancers. A leading BHRT Expert Dr. Devaki Berkson recently wrote: ***We have had over 15 reanalyses of the ill-fated WRONG first Women's Health Initiative (WHI) that show that:***

- Estrogen protects breast tissue in healthy women against getting breast cancer.
- And if you are or were on estrogen replacement for an average of 5 years, and you did get breast cancer, it's most often a

"better player" (less aggressive) and you most likely die less from it (statistically reduced fatality incidence).

If you would like to hear me interview Dr. Gary Donovitz several years ago regarding BHRT and breast cancer it can be viewed on You Tube, https://youtu.be/1COAAex_bTY?si=3nQW8aSvzKMNBROD

After dissecting study after study, the truth remains that estrogen does not cause breast cancer.

Bioidentical Testosterone Replacement Therapy: Not Just for Men

Many people assume testosterone to be an exclusively "male" hormone. While it's true that testosterone is the primary a male, not a female sex hormone, the assumption that it's not crucial for optimal women's health is incorrect.

Our ovaries produce both testosterone and estradiol. These hormones decline naturally with age or with surgical menopause may make this happen sooner and we just don't feel well. Many times, it is hard to put our finger on why we don't feel as good as we did 10-15 years ago. Once we do the initial blood panel you can clearly see the reason. Many times, the estradiol and testosterone levels are so low, they can't be measured at the lab.

As I have alluded to several times already, bioidentical testosterone therapy is not only beneficial for aging men; it's also proven to substantially help women experiencing menopause, as critical testosterone levels decline in women during this phase of life just as they do in the aging male body over time. However, the drop-off of testosterone levels in women during menopause tends to occur more rapidly and therefore with more immediate and severe resulting symptoms than the drip-drip-drip decline in testosterone seen in the aging male body.

While women typically have just one-tenth to one-twelfth the circulating testosterone as men, it's nonetheless a vital component of women's hormone systems, playing a central role in the regulation of numerous physiological processes.

The recognition of the massive therapeutic upside of bioidentical testosterone therapy for menopausal women has grown immensely over the past decade or so.

Dr. James Simon, MD, participating in an expert panel discussion on the role of testosterone therapy in anti-aging medicine for women, published in the medical journal OBG Management [27], had the following to say in its value:

> *"Much of the beneficial data for testosterone's use is for sexual function in postmenopausal women. Female sexual dysfunction is highly prevalent among women during the post menopause.* ***Androgen levels progressively decrease throughout adult life in all women, so the postmenopausal additional lack of estrogen has a recognized effect on genitourinary* health****. There is evidence that* ***the insufficiency of androgens as well as estrogens after menopause can lead to genitourinary symptoms*** *of menopause (GSM).* ***Testosterone also is used for increasing strength, lean muscle mass, bone mineral density, and sense of well-being****."*

("Genitourinary" is a medical term relating to the genital and urinary organs.)

Another participant in the panel of expert, Dr. Rebecca Glaser, MD, reports using testosterone therapy for her menopausal patients to treat a cornucopia of menopause-related symptoms, including:

- Anxiety
- Irritability
- Fatigue
- Decreased libido, sexual activity, or pleasure
- Vasomotor instability
- Bone loss
- Decreased muscle strength
- Insomnia

- Urinary symptoms
- Incontinence
- Changes in cognition
- Memory loss
- Vaginal atrophy and dryness
- Joint and muscle pain

The widespread therapeutic applications of bioidentical testosterone for women are not shocking; just like men, women have androgen receptors located throughout their bodies that require nourishment in the form of circulating testosterone to function at their peak.

You might be asking yourself by this point, "If bioidentical testosterone therapy is so effective for women experiencing menopause, why have I never heard about it until now? And why has no healthcare practitioner ever recommended it to me?"

These are excellent questions that deserve answers for the sake of women's anti-aging health. It has been suggested, with good evidence to back up the assertion, by many frontline doctors and researchers, that gender bias has for far too long played a role in the historical lack of appropriate attention paid to bioidentical testosterone therapy for women.

Here is Dr. Angela DeRosa, founder of the Hormone Health Institute in Scottsdale Arizona on the issue of gender bias in the field of hormone healthcare, via the International Journal of Pharmaceutical Compounding [28]:

> ***"Gender bias within hormone replacement therapy has been prevalent for decades*** *and the circumstances continue to worsen with existing guidelines, 'expert' consensus statements, and a 'newly released report' from the National Academies of Sciences, Engineering, and Medicine (NASEM)...*
>
> *Overall* ***gender bias... is highly prevalent in medical research and care of women; and in particular the lack of commercially***

> ***available U.S. Food and Drug Administration (FDA)-approved testosterone products for women...***
>
> ***Much of the research [on testosterone therapy]*** *to date has focused on men, with information extrapolated to women, even though this is physiologically and medically inappropriate."*

In other words, you can't find answers to questions that are never asked, for example: what are the anti-aging health benefits of bioidentical testosterone replacement therapy for women experiencing menopause?

Fortunately, the tides have turned in recent years in terms of studying the application of bioidentical testosterone in women's healthcare. Let's take a brief look here at some of the latest, exciting research in the field.

One exciting study brought to light in 2021 involved the administration of BHRT with bioidentical testosterone pellets to over 2,000 menopausal and postmenopausal women, who were then followed for a period of nine years to assess the development (or lack thereof) of breast cancer compared to the general public.

Here are the results, via Business Wire [29]:

> *"Women who took testosterone via hormone pellets as part of bioidentical hormone replacement therapy (BHRT) had a* ***35.5% lower incidence of invasive breast cancer*** *compared to expected age-adjusted Surveillance Epidemiology and End Results (SEER) rates, according to a new retrospective study."*

Now, I don't have to tell you that a 35.5% reduction in breast cancer risk from a *single* therapeutic intervention, bioidentical testosterone pellets for menopausal women is a godsend for the millions of Americans affected by this devastating disease each year. It's these kinds of studies, which make the longstanding denial of the benefits of BHRT for menopausal women impossible to maintain, that get me jazzed to deliver this critical anti-aging therapy to my patients. We are fortunate in our community that we have two medical oncologists that have dove into the research and refer breast cancer patients to LowTE Florida after they have completed their treatment. They appreciate the quality of life benefits as well as the potential risks reduction.

Dr. Gary Donovitz, the co-author of the cited study, explained that "given the way testosterone functions within the body, breast cancer prevention is an unsurprising but crucial addition to the corpus of research on hormone optimization, and this study adds to our knowledge of testosterone's vital importance to women's health."

He went on to add: "this study reaffirms that hormone imbalances are an urgent medical condition for women, and that optimizing hormones responsibly cannot just improve quality of life, but actually prevent disease."

In its "guide to prescribing testosterone for women in primary care," the British Journal of General Practice [30] lauded the extremely wide-ranging and now well-documented benefits of bioidentical testosterone as a holistic approach to menopausal women's hormone care:

> ***"Numerous studies have shown that adding testosterone to hormonal therapy can improve sexual function and general wellbeing among women during their menopause.*** *A recent systematic review and meta-analysis of testosterone treatment in women has provided robust support for a trial of testosterone in women when clinically indicated.* ***In postmenopausal women, testosterone supplementation improved several domains of sexual response, including sexual desire, pleasure, arousal, orgasm, and self-image.***
>
> ***It has also been shown to have additional benefits including*** *the improvement of urogenital, psychological, and somatic symptoms, an* ***increase in bone density, and enhancement of cognitive performance when combined with estrogen as part of HRT.*** *Many women notice that* ***taking testosterone improves their mood, concentration, motivation, and energy levels.*** *"*

If you're a woman going through the trying time of menopause or post menopause, I need not elaborate further on the demonstrable value of this therapy for improving cognition, enhancing energy levels, and restoring female sexual health and libido.

The Hormone X-Factor: Bioidentical Progesterone

Progesterone, though often overlooked, is another vital female sex hormone that supports a healthy menstrual cycle as well as healthy pregnancy in women by helping to ready the endometrium (uterus lining) to implant and nurture a fertilized egg.

Because it often takes a back seat to estrogen therapy, some might colorfully call progesterone the "red-headed stepchild" of hormone care. However, the need for bioidentical progesterone therapy in combination with bioidentical estrogen therapy is never overlooked at my LowTE Florida office.

Progesterone must exist within a certain ratio to estrogen in the female body for optimal health. Without a proper balance between progesterone and estrogen (for those with a uterus) serious health consequences can emerge, including cancer.

In an earlier chapter, we cited research published in the Journal of Obstetrics and Gynecology [31] demonstrating conclusively that the concurrent administration of progesterone and estrogen virtually eliminated the risk of endometrial hyperplasia, the medical term for unhealthy thickening of the uterine lining very likely to lead to cancer if left untreated, often seen in female patients receiving estrogen therapy without accompanying progesterone:

> *"Among the 1385 patients with valid biopsy data, endometrial hyperplasia developed in 20% in the conjugated estrogens-treated group and < or = 1% in each of the four conjugated estrogens/medroxyprogesterone acetate-treated groups. The incidence of endometrial hyperplasia did not differ significantly between any of the conjugated estrogens/medroxyprogesterone*

> *acetate regimens. However,* ***none of the patients receiving the two higher medroxyprogesterone acetate dosages (groups B and D) had endometrial hyperplasia.*** *"*

It is for these reasons and more that I administer bioidentical progesterone (never the synthetic form, progestin, which can cause more health problems than it solves) alongside bioidentical estrogen in my menopausal patients.

The clinical literature further indicates that naturally occurring, bioidentical progesterone is safer and more effective for use in therapy than the commonly used synthetic form of progesterone progestin, as explained by way of 2018 research published in Climacteric [32], followed by a call from the medical journal for a "regulatory agency-approved [hormone therapy] with naturally occurring [estradiol]/[progesterone]":

> ***"[Bioidentical progesterone] used in [hormone therapy] prevents endometrial hyperplasia from estrogens while helping relieve vasomotor symptoms and improving quality-of-life measures.*** *Additionally, risk of* ***venous thromboembolism and breast cancer does not appear to increase with use of [bioidentical progesterone] plus estrogens as shown with synthetic progestins plus*** *estrogens in large observations studies, and* ***no detrimental effects of [bioidentical progesterone] in HT have been found on outcomes related to cardiovascular disease or cognition.***
>
> *A regulatory agency-approved [hormone therapy] with naturally occurring [estradiol]/[progesterone] could be an option for the millions of women who desire a bioidentical product."*

Several of the more advanced and up to date hormone research scientists such as Dr. Lindsey Berkson are promoting progesterone for women without a uterus and even men. She writes in her sub-stack article on Progesterone:

"Progesterone is constantly produced in middle-aged humans in lots of places, such as: Six places in the brain, in the coronary artery, in the gut wall, in the lining of the lungs, to protect multiple tissues - in both genders. I could go on and on.

Progesterone is made globally (meaning all over our bodies) because progesterone has so many uses. Progesterone's signals have so many protective actions.

We are just beginning to appreciate the tip of the iceberg of what hormones do in general, and progesterone in particular.

Progesterone signals our calming nervous system, our parasympathetic nervous system."

So, if you are a woman without a uterus and you would like to net the benefits of progesterone therapy just let me know!

Imagine my surprise when my brother's oncologist prescribed progesterone (granted, a synthetic version) to help with his lung cancer treatment! Dr. Berkson is on to something!

Again, because I am committed to delivering to my patients nothing but the best, informed by the latest cutting-edge science, at my LowTE Florida office, I exclusively use bioidentical progesterone, never synthetic progestin in the provision of BHRT and they reap the superior benefits.

I have found it interesting that many pharmacists don't understand the huge differences between synthetic progestins and bioidentical progesterone. I delivered a presentation to a group of over 200 pharmacists a few years ago sharing the differences. I was surprised, they were on the edges of their seats and had lots of good questions. I was afraid they were going to roast this Nurse Practitioner!

HRT Success Stories for Women at LowTE Florida

Success stories of my female patients visiting LowTE Florida office since I first opened my doors in 1994 that's 30 years' worth of optimized hormones and restored lives are plenty.

Here my patient Suzanna E. shares her recent experience via Yelp:

> *"I've started going to LowTE for the first time on January 26, 2023. The results 6 weeks later were very noticeable. I've lost 14 pounds with these hormones pellets while remaining on my rigorous exercise schedule during the week.* ***I've been in this rigorous gym program for one-year last month in February and didn't lose a pound until I started taking these hormone pellets*****. My energy levels are back. I feel like I'm thinking clearer, and everything is much easier for me to accomplish now. I feel like I'm getting my spunky self-back finally. It's been a journey, thank you so much for everything. I highly recommend the hormone pellets. It changes your life."*

*This is an extremely common phenomenon: you go to the gym, work your tail off, eat right, yet still don't see the results you are looking for in terms of greater energy, weight loss, etc. The issue that Suzanna, like many women, had, was fundamentally hormonal. It wasn't until we got her hormones optimized with an individualized treatment plan that everything, including her weight loss goals, fell into place.

And, via Google, my patient Patricia N. shares her own journey to better hormone health with LowTE Florida:

> *"The hormone therapy program offered by LowTE Florida is top-notch. The program is tailored to the unique needs of each patient, and the team takes the time to explain every aspect of the treatment plan. The results have been nothing short of amazing. I feel healthier, more energetic, and more focused than I have in years.*

> *One of the things I appreciate most about LowTE Florida is their commitment to ongoing education and training. They stay up to date on the latest advances in hormone therapy and are always looking for ways to improve their services. It's clear that they take their work seriously and are passionate about helping their patients achieve optimal health.*
>
> *I highly recommend LowTE Florida to anyone seeking hormone therapy."*

Finally, LowTE Florida patient Laura R. offers this beautifully succinct review via Google:

> *"I have been a grateful patient here for years. After searching for the right fit in my change of life Carolyn brought more to my wellness than I ever imagined. This is the most comfortable and welcoming medical practice I have ever experienced. I am a loyal client and I would follow her anywhere. She is always available and generous with her time and knowledge. It's a thoroughly positive experience."*

There are simply too many of these accounts to share here. I encourage you, if you are interested in unfiltered reviews from real patients, to simply Google "LowTE Florida." A plethora of bona fide review sites Facebook, Yelp, Google, etc. will pop up with more real-life testimonials than you can dream of.

References

[1] Faubion, S., Enders, F., et al. (2023). Impact of Menopause Symptoms on Women in the Workplace. Mayo Clinic Proceedings. https://www.mayoclinicproceedings.org/pb-assets/Health%20Advance/journals/jmcp/JMCP4097_proof.pdf

[2] Gordon, Deb. (2021). 73% Of Women Don't Treat Their Menopause Symptoms, New Survey Shows. Forbes. https://www.forbes.com/sites/debgordon/2021/07/13/73-of-women-dont-treat-their-menopause-symptoms-new-survey-shows/

[3] The Lancet. (2022). Attitudes towards menopause: time for change. The Lancet. https://www.thelancet.com/journals/lancet/article/PIIS0140-6736(22)01099-6/fulltext

[4] Kotz, Deborah. (2009). Bioidentical Hormones: Safer For Hot Flashes Than HRT? U.S. News and World Report https://health.usnews.com/health-news/family-health/articles/2009/03/25/bioidentical-hormones-safer-for-hot-flashes-than-hrt

[5] Polo-Kantola, P., Erkkola, R., et al. (1998). When does estrogen replacement therapy improve sleep quality? American Journal of Obstetrics and Gynecology. https://pubmed.ncbi.nlm.nih.gov/9609575/

[6] Gambacciani, M. and Levancini, M. (2014). Hormone replacement therapy and the prevention of postmenopausal osteoporosis. Menopause Review. https://www.ncbi.nlm.nih.gov/pmc/articles/PMC4520366/

[7] Xiao-Ping, Y. and Reckelhoff, J. (2011). Estrogen, hormonal replacement therapy and cardiovascular disease. Current Opinion in Nephrology and Hypertension. https://www.ncbi.nlm.nih.gov/pmc/articles/PMC3123884/

[8] McCubbin, J., Helfer, S., et al. (2002). Blood pressure control and hormone replacement therapy in postmenopausal women at risk for coronary heart disease. American Heart Journal. https://pubmed.ncbi.nlm.nih.gov/11923810/

[9] Denke, M. (1995). Effects of continuous combined hormone-replacement therapy on lipid levels in hypercholesterolemic postmenopausal women. The American Journal of Medicine. https://pubmed.ncbi.nlm.nih.gov/7598139/

[10] Redberg, R., Nishino, M. et al. (2000). Long-term estrogen replacement therapy is associated with improved exercise capacity in postmenopausal women without known coronary artery disease. American Heart Journal. https://pubmed.ncbi.nlm.nih.gov/10740161/

[11] Hogervorst, E., craig, J., et al. (2022). Cognition and mental health in menopause: A review. Best Practice & Research Clinical Obstetrics & Gynaecology. https://pubmed.ncbi.nlm.nih.gov/34969617/

[12] Shors, T and Leuner, B. (2003). Estrogen-mediated effects on depression and memory formation in females. The Journal of Affective Disorders. https://www.ncbi.nlm.nih.gov/pmc/articles/PMC3374589/

[13] Boyle, C., Cyrus, A., et al. (2021). Estrogen, brain structure, and cognition in postmenopausal women. Human Brain Mapping. https://www.ncbi.nlm.nih.gov/pmc/articles/PMC7721237/

[14] Dutt, P., Chaudhary, S., et al. (2013). Oral Health and Menopause: A Comprehensive Review on Current Knowledge and Associated Dental Management. Annals of Medical and Health Sciences Research. https://www.ncbi.nlm.nih.gov/pmc/articles/PMC3793432/

[15] Paganini-Hill, A. (1995). The benefits of estrogen replacement therapy on oral health. The Leisure World cohort. Archives of Internal Medicine. https://pubmed.ncbi.nlm.nih.gov/7487257/

[17] Chmouliovsky, L., Habicht, F., et al. (1999). Beneficial effect of hormone replacement therapy on weight loss in obese menopausal women. Maturitas. https://pubmed.ncbi.nlm.nih.gov/10515671/

[17] Bartosch, J. (2023). Why am I gaining weight so fast during menopause? And will hormone therapy help? University of Chicago Medicine. https://www.uchicagomedicine.org/forefront/womens-health-articles/menopause-weight-gain-hormone-therapy

[18] Roman-Blas, J., Castañeda, S., et al. (2009). Osteoarthritis associated with estrogen deficiency. Arthritis Research & Therapy. https://www.ncbi.nlm.nih.gov/pmc/articles/PMC2787275/

[19] Chidi-Ogbolu, K. and Baar, K. (2018) Effect of Estrogen on Musculoskeletal Performance and Injury Risk. Frontiers in Physiology. https://www.ncbi.nlm.nih.gov/pmc/articles/PMC6341375/

[20] Cappelletti, M. and Wallen, K. (2016). Increasing women's sexual desire: The comparative effectiveness of estrogens and androgens. Hormones and Behavior. https://www.ncbi.nlm.nih.gov/pmc/articles/PMC4720522/

[21] Sarrel, P. (2000). Effects of hormone replacement therapy on sexual psychophysiology and behavior in post menopause. Journal of Women s Health & Gender-Based Medicine. https://pubmed.ncbi.nlm.nih.gov/10695871/

[22] Sehl, M. and Ganz, P. (2018). Potential Mechanisms of Age Acceleration Caused by Estrogen Deprivation: Do Endocrine Therapies Carry the Same Risks? JNCI Cancer Spectrum. https://www.ncbi.nlm.nih.gov/pmc/articles/PMC6649786/

[23] Paganini-Hill, A., Corrada, M. et al. (2018). Increased longevity in older users of postmenopausal estrogen therapy: the Leisure World Cohort Study. Menopause. https://www.ncbi.nlm.nih.gov/pmc/articles/PMC7219089/

[24] Zubialde, J., Lawler, F., et al. (1993). Estimated gains in life expectancy with use of postmenopausal estrogen therapy: a decision analysis. The Journal of Family Practice. https://pubmed.ncbi.nlm.nih.gov/8454973/

[25] Zethraeus, N., Johannesson, M. (1997). The impact of hormone replacement therapy on quality of life and willingness to pay. British Journal of Obstetrics and Gynecology. https://pubmed.ncbi.nlm.nih.gov/9332999/

[26] Lee, S., Cho, M. et al. (2020). The 2020 Menopausal Hormone Therapy Guidelines. Journal of Menopausal Medicine. https://www.ncbi.nlm.nih.gov/pmc/articles/PMC7475284/

[27] Karram, M., Glaser, R., et al. (2021). Testosterone supplementation in women: When, why, and how. OBG Management. https://www.belmarpharmasolutions.com/wp-content/uploads/2021/07/OBGM_0321_Roundtable_FINAL.pdf?utm_source=Pardot&utm_medium=email&utm_campaign=20210820_WpAPM_BEL-PRO_OFU-ICYMI-Reminder

[28] DeRosa, A. (2021). Gender Bias in the Treatment of Menopausal Women: I am Hot as Hell and Not Going to Take It Anymore, Part 2. International Journal of Pharmaceutical Compounding. https://www.belmarpharmasolutions.com/wp-content/uploads/2021/01/Im-Hot-As-Hell....Part-II-IJCP.pdf?utm_source=Pardot&utm_medium=email&utm_campaign=20210820_WpAPM_BEL-PRO_OFU-ICYMI-Reminder

[29] Business Wire. (2021). Study: Testosterone Pellet Therapy Reduces Breast Cancer Incidence in Women. Business Wire. https://www.business wire.com/news/home/20210511005434/en/Study-Testosterone-Pellet-Therapy-Reduces-Breast-Cancer-Incidence-in-Women

[30] Scott, A. and Newsom, L. (2020). Should we be prescribing testosterone to perimenopausal and menopausal women? A guide to prescribing testosterone for women in primary care. British Journal of General Practice. https://www.ncbi.nlm.nih.gov/pmc/articles/PMC7098532/

[31] Woodruff, J., et al. (1994). Incidence of endometrial hyperplasia in postmenopausal women taking. American Journal of Obstetrics and Gynecology. https://www.ajog.org/article/S0002-9378(94)70129-6/fulltext

[32] Mirkin, S. (2018). Evidence on the use of progesterone in menopausal hormone therapy. Climacteric. https://pubmed.ncbi.nlm.nih.gov/29630427/

Chapter VII
Bioidentical Hormone Replacement for Men

Testosterone, put succinctly, is the hormone that makes men *"men,"* producing all the dimorphic secondary sex characteristics associated with masculinity, as compared to femininity: higher muscle mass, greater physical strength, thicker skin, denser, larger bones, the male genitalia, male hip structure, sperm production, etc.

Via the United States Institute of Medicine [1]:

> *"Testosterone and its metabolites play a crucial role in the health and development of the male....*
>
> *During puberty,* ***testosterone is required for the development of male secondary sexual characteristics, stimulation of sexual behavior and function, and initiation of sperm production****....*
>
> *In adult males,* ***testosterone is involved in maintaining muscle mass and strength, fat distribution, bone mass, red blood cell production, male hair pattern, libido and potency, and spermatogenesis."***

The testes produce the bulk of testosterone circulating in men's bodies, although smaller amounts are also excreted by the adrenal glands located above the kidneys.

Without optimal levels of testosterone on hand to nourish the cells, tissues, and organs, a clinical testosterone deficiency develops into an anti-aging health challenge, that is unfortunately widespread among older men. Without replacing dropping testosterone levels, including through bioidentical hormone replacement therapy, achieving peak health in all aspects of life (mental, emotional, and physical) is impossible.

Stats on Age-Related Declines in Male Testosterone Levels

On average, although individual physiology, genetic, and environmental factors weigh heavily into the equation, **men tend to lose approximately 1% of their total free testosterone every year (!)** following peak concentrations of the male sex hormone achieved in their late teens or early twenties. (I'll explain the important difference between "total," "free," and "bound" testosterone in short order.)

> *"Levels of plasma testosterone increase in males [to] reach normal male adult levels of 10 to 35 nmol/L (approximately 300 to 1,000 ng/dL) by about age 17. Levels of bioavailable testosterone remain level until men are in their 30s to 40s then the levels begin to decline about 1.2 percent per year," reports the U.S. Institute of Medicine.*

Work published in Sports Health[2] further explains the aging-related decline seen in male testosterone levels over time:

> *"It is well understood that testosterone levels decline with age. Around **20% of 60-year-olds and 50% of 80-year-olds exhibit total serum testosterone levels below the normal range** for young men. **Such low levels are commonly associated with erectile dysfunction, loss of libido, muscle weakness, lower bone mass, and frailty."***

Far from being a mere detriment to men's quality of life, low testosterone levels are deadly if left untreated.

To that effect, a brand-new 2024 landmark Annals of Internal Medicine [3] meta-analysis (meaning a synthesis of the findings of related clinical studies in order to identify through-lines and ultimately arrive at a more robust conclusion) found a significant direct correlation between testosterone levels and all-cause mortality (AKA death), with a particular positive relationship between low T and heart disease:

"Nine studies provided individual participant data (IPD) (255 830 participant-years). Eleven studies provided summary estimates (n = 24 109). Two-stage random-effects IPD meta-analyses found that ***men with baseline testosterone concentrations below 7.4 nmol/L (<213 ng/dL), LH concentrations above 10 IU/L, or estradiol concentrations below 5.1 pmol/L had higher all-cause mortality****, and* ***those with testosterone concentrations below 5.3 nmol/L (<153 ng/dL) had higher CVD mortality risk****. Lower SHBG concentration was associated with lower all-cause mortality (median for quintile 1 [Q1] vs. Q5, 20.6 vs. 68.3 nmol/L; adjusted hazard ratio [HR], 0.85 [95% CI, 0.77 to 0.95]) and lower CVD mortality (adjusted HR, 0.81 [CI, 0.65 to 1.00]) .... Men with DHT concentrations below 0.59 nmol/L had increased risk for incident CVD events...*

Men with low testosterone, high LH, or very low estradiol concentrations had increased all-cause mortality."

The meta-analysis also, importantly, found a positive relationship between higher sex hormone binding globulin (SHBG) levels and death, which is not surprising because, as we will explore now, SHBG "binds" otherwise free testosterone, rendering it biologically inactive and essentially useless in terms of feeding the tissues and organs the potent male sex hormone they crave.

As promised, let's unpack the distinctions between the different forms of testosterone we alluded to previously:

- Free testosterone
- Bound testosterone
- Total testosterone

The first kind, free testosterone is the kind of testosterone you want and need. This is because free testosterone is bioactive, meaning it goes to work on the tissues and organs that need its help. Bound testosterone, on the other hand, is so named because it is "bound" to one of two types of protein and therefore ineffective from the perspective of sex hormone optimization.

In fact, the overwhelming majority of testosterone in the blood supply is "bound" rather than "free," an issue that can be remedied through BHRT.

> "Approximately 98 percent of testosterone circulates in the blood is bound to protein, of which approximately 60 percent is bound weakly to albumin and other proteins and 40 percent is bound with higher binding affinity to sex hormone binding globulin (SHBG)," notes the U.S. Institute of Medicine. That renders just 2% of all the endogenous testosterone in the body bioavailable, or "free"!"

This nuanced distinction between the three types of testosterones presents thorny clinical dilemmas to anti-aging healthcare practitioners, as explained via Sports Health:

> ***"Defining who is truly hypogonadal remains somewhat controversial. The most common method is the measurement of total testosterone,*** *which is reported by some authors as low when serum concentrations are less than 200 ng/dL regardless of age.* ***Total testosterone, however, includes a significant portion that is bound to sex hormone–binding globulin, which is biologically inactive,*** *leading some authors to suggest* ***measuring bioavailable, or 'free,' testosterone as a more accurate reflection of the hormone's active concentration.*** *Furthermore, because of variability in assays, diurnal and situational variation, and a range of normal values, it is difficult to make a diagnosis of hypogonadism on the basis of a laboratory value alone. Thus, most authors suggest combining a low testosterone level with clinical symptoms such as loss of libido, erectile dysfunction, and loss of muscle mass or sarcopenia for an accurate diagnosis."*

Obviously, based on the information above, expertly differentiating between total, bound, and free testosterone while interpreting blood panel results, your symptoms, and vital metrics in a holistic, integrated diagnostic process is critical to accurately assess any hormone deficiency.

An in-depth analysis of all these data points is also, naturally, critical to develop an effective therapeutic strategy accordingly yet another illustration of the importance of working with a seasoned hormone expert like the ones we house in our LowTE Florida clinical team.

The Proven Benefits of Bioidentical Testosterone for Men

As explained below via Sports Health, the logic behind the application of BHRT for men with low T is both sound and well-supported, with a long history of use in clinical practice going back decades (although it was historically mostly limited to the world of athletic competition):

> *"While* ***the performance-enhancing effects of testosterone have been known in athletic populations since the 1950s****, there has recently been a considerable amount of work investigating its role in aging populations. The justification behind this work is logical:* ***Many of the more apparent changes of aging, such as loss of muscle and bone mass, libido, and energy, are often the inverse of what is reported in testosterone users****... Replacing testosterone in an older population may lead to reversal of some of these negative effects."*

The power of bioidentical hormones is not speculative; I've seen the transformations in my male patients up close thousands of times over.

Accordingly, I can say with confidence that, for the vast majority of men with documented testosterone deficiencies, **there is no one anti-aging medical intervention more broadly effective** at restoring vitality, rebuilding lost muscle mass, re-strengthening bones, clearing up mental health difficulties, enhancing physical performance, supercharging libido, improving overall quality of life, lengthening lifespan, etc. **than**

BHRT with bioidentical testosterone pellets. No pharmaceutical drug, no surgery, no laser therapy, no supplement regimen (although, as we'll discuss in a later chapter, supplementation is also a powerful anti-aging tool when used in combination with hormone therapy). Nothing.

Nothing outshines the mighty bioidentical hormone pellet for reversing the negative health effects of low T. So, if you are experiencing brain fog, erectile dysfunction, low energy, or any of the myriad and often non-specific signs of testosterone deficiency that we'll explore coming up, especially if you're over 35, and your primary care doctor isn't investigating your testosterone levels and developing a protocol to increase them, if necessary, it's time to look elsewhere, like LowTE Florida for expert help.

First, before we get into the definitive list of low T symptoms and the benefits of BHRT benefits for men experiencing them, let's discuss male testosterone levels, what constitutes a testosterone deficiency, and the optimal levels that we achieve at LowTE Florida through BHRT:

- Testosterone levels **below 300 nanograms per deciliter (ng/dL)** are considered **deficient**
- Testosterone levels **between 300-1,000 nanograms per deciliter (ng/dL) are healthy** (however, I prefer to see my patients get into the upper range of that scale, much closer to 1,000 ng/dL than 300 ng/dL)

A simple, inexpensive, in-and-out blood test, which I perform for all my new patients as standard operating procedure, can determine your baseline testosterone levels.

Accompanying low levels of testosterone, my patients often present with the following symptoms:

- Loss of libido (sex drive)
- Erectile dysfunction
- Shrinking testicles
- Infertility
- Enlarged prostate (triggering urination issues)
- Sleep disturbances (insomnia)

- Difficulty concentrating
- Loss of interest in former passions
- Gynecomastia (male breast development)
- Anxiety
- Depression
- Chronic fatigue
- Loss of muscle mass
- Osteoporosis (bone weakening)

...among many, many others!

I have mentioned this before, but it bears repeating as you can see, these symptoms associated with low T are wide-ranging and mostly non-specific, particularly the ones not related to sexual health, meaning they could potentially be tied to any number of chronic or acute health conditions other than a hormone deficit.

"There are many signs and symptoms of Low Testosterone. Some are more closely related to Low-T levels (specific signs and symptoms). Others may not necessarily be linked (non-specific signs and symptoms)," notes the Urology Care Foundation [4]. "Non-specific symptoms are those that may or may not be linked to [testosterone deficiency] ... Having any one of the specific or non-specific symptoms may not mean that you have [testosterone deficiency]."

You may be surprised to hear that the number one reason men seek out TRT is fatigue. One would think it would be low libido or ED, but no, I see it daily when doing the initial consultation.

This is, again, why seeking out the expert guidance of a seasoned team of practitioners (like that which you'll discover at LowTE Florida) is vital.

The expertise of *general* medicine practitioners, while they are important and, in fact, critical frontline healthcare providers whom I would never disparage, is just that: *general*. They are not specifically or extensively trained in the practice of hormone optimization. As a result, they may, and often do, misattribute the symptoms of hormone deficiency to another health condition, resulting in a misdiagnosis and, unfortunately, a lack of recovery for the patient. I spend my days trying to dispel the myths and misinformation that many of my patients are getting from friends, family, doctors, and the internet. Unfortunately, we have learned over time that if traditional doctors are not "up on hormone therapy they are down on it". Please find an enlightened and educated provider.

This doesn't need to be the situation in modern medicine. We now have within reach, even for patients of modest means, the diagnostic and therapeutic tools to easily and inexpensively identify and reverse testosterone deficiencies. I know this because I perform this work at LowTE Florida every day of the week.

Pivoting now to the benefits of BHRT with bioidentical testosterone for men with low T, should we find through testing that your levels are sub-optimal, my colleague (and a renowned leader in the hormone optimization space), Director of the Laboratory for Andrology Research at McNair Medical Institute, Baylor College of Medicine, Dr. Mohit Khera, had the following to say on the topic in a January 2024 conversation with Dr. Rachel Rubin, published via Medscape [5]:

> ***"There's a profound effect on quality of life for many men who initiate testosterone therapy****. The typical man is older; remember that roughly 60% of patients who come in who have low testosterone levels will have metabolic syndrome, diabetes, or obesity. That syndrome is there. He now has erectile dysfunction, low libido, and some depression. He has increased fat deposition, and decreased muscle mass. He's now having some difficulty in his relationship with his partner because he cannot engage in sexual activity, so he is stressed. When you put these patients on testosterone, many of them could see a significant improvement in their energy. Fat deposition declines and muscle mass improves. They work out, and their erectile function can improve, particularly if they are using a PDE-5 inhibitor in combination therapy.*
>
> (note: PDE-5 inhibitors are Cialis, Viagra and Levitra) ***If you watch them over time, these patients are extremely appreciative when***

> ***they come in, thanking you for making a profound impact on their quality of life."***

(Coming up shortly, we'll get into testimonials of health transformations from my real-life patients at LowTE Florida who have been kind enough to share their experiences.)

What follows is a handful (but by no measure all) of the benefits, backed by research, that my male patients at LowTE Florida reap from BHRT with bioidentical testosterone.

Bioidentical Testosterone Improves Cardiovascular Health and Heart Function in Men

The cells of the heart and blood vessels are replete with androgen receptors (ARs), through which they interact with testosterone, which in turn exerts protective effects on the cardiovascular system.

Here are the results of a massive, comprehensive study of over 83,000 male U.S. armed forces veterans, published via the European Heart Journal [6], titled "Normalization of testosterone level is associated with reduced incidence of myocardial infarction and mortality in men":

> *"We retrospectively examined 83,010 male veterans with documented low [testosterone] levels...*
>
> *In this large observational cohort with extended follow-up, normalization of [testosterone] levels after TRT was associated with a significant reduction in all-cause mortality, [heart attack], and stroke."*

The differences between the experimental group (the veterans with documented low testosterone who received therapy) and the control group (the ones with documented low T whose deficiency was not treated) were stark. Dare I say, they were *shocking.*

The results of the study show that the American veterans with low T who received therapy and restored their testosterone to healthy levels had a whopping **56% reduction in all-cause mortality (death)**, a **36% reduction in strokes**, and a **24% reduction in heart attacks following treatment**.

I challenge you to find anywhere in the clinical literature a single medical intervention for men with low testosterone demonstrated to achieve anything remotely approaching a 56% reduction in all-cause mortality. (Feel free to look but let me save you some time with a spoiler alert: none exist.)

Bioidentical Testosterone Relieves Depression and Anxiety in Men

It's no secret that society conditions men to hesitate to talk about (let alone seek professional help for) mental health conditions like depression and anxiety.

Yet, whether male mental health is publicly discussed or not, the rates of such afflictions are astronomically high in the United States, due to a toxic brew of environmental contaminants, the chronic stress induced by hectic modern life, poor diet, insufficient sleep and, yes, untreated testosterone deficiencies.

If you live in America in the 21st century, statistics predict that you either know personally or are yourself a man who has been impacted by mental health conditions.

And hormones play a large, underappreciated role in our mental health epidemic.

The brain and nervous system are chockfull of androgen receptors. In the presence of optimal levels of testosterone, they are nourished and thrive consequently. Deprived of testosterone, as in the case of low T, the cells and tissues of the central nervous system fall into disrepair and mental health suffers.

I can't tell you how many men have come through my LowTE Florida office doors with complaints of mood disorders, depression, and anxiety, many of whom have previously sought (through their primary care doctors or psychiatrists or other non-hormone specialists) conventional treatment (like serotonin reuptake inhibitors, or SSRIs, for example).

The overwhelming majority of these men experienced no lasting relief with those treatments.

But, once I've tested their blood, we find their testosterone levels in the basement. We then treat them accordingly with bioidentical testosterone pellets, and, *voila*, within a matter of months, if not weeks, they're back to their happy, productive, engaged, motivated selves.

Consider the findings below of a meta-analysis of almost 30 clinical trials, examining the depression-alleviating benefits of testosterone administered to nearly 2,000 clinically depressed men, published in 2018 by the Journal of the American Medical Association [7]:

> *"Random-effects meta-analysis of 27 RCTs including 1890 men suggested that* ***testosterone treatment is associated with a significant reduction in depressive symptoms compared with placebo...***
>
> *In the most conservative bias scenario, testosterone treatment remained significant whenever dosages greater than 0.5 g/wk were administered...*
>
> *Testosterone treatment appears to be effective and efficacious in reducing depressive symptoms in men, particularly when higher-dosage regimens were applied in carefully selected samples."*

Bioidentical Testosterone Enhances Cognition in Men

A benefit related to improved mental health following testosterone replacement therapy in men but critical is cognition -the ability to interpret, process, and store information, otherwise known more simply in common parlance as "thinking."

It's well-known that a deterioration in cognition, or clear thinking, often goes hand-in-hand with the aging process. You may have seen this play out with an older relative.

However, it doesn't have to be this way. There is no divine decree or biological imperative that, as you age, you therefore lose the capacity to reason with all the same mental faculties that you had in your 20s, 30s, or 40s.

Cognitive decline, including that caused by neurodegenerative diseases like Alzheimer's, Parkinson's, etc., is a serious and growing public health threat. So far, conventional medicine has been unable to find a "silver bullet" prevention or cure.

As an exceedingly complex phenomenon (the human brain being the most complex organ ever studied) there are many variables that contribute to cognitive decline, but hormone deficiencies and all their downstream effects like increased inflammation are a **major** factor, and arguably the most important of them all.

I submit to you, future LowTE Florida patient of mine, that hormones (testosterone, specifically, for men) have been woefully neglected in the search for the anti-aging Holy Grail when it comes to preventing cognitive decline.

And the consequences of neglected hormone health are devastating for our collective cognitive health.

The researchers in one landmark study, for instance, using data from National Health and Nutrition Examination Survey and published in the journal Frontiers in Aging Neuroscience [8], led their introduction with the following flurry of devastating facts:

> *"Cognitive performance, including memory, attention, language and visuospatial ability, declines with age. As life expectancy increases, age-related cognitive decline may be a great health challenge for older adults, cognitive health has become a major public health issue for the aging population in the United States.*

The process from cognitive decline to dementia is continuous and irreversible. ***In America, approximately 5.1 million people have dementia, and that is expected to double by 2050. The financial burden of dementia has exceeded the costs of cardiovascular and cancer diseases.*** *The global cost of dementia was $957.56 billion in 2015 and is projected to reach $9.12 trillion by 2050.* ***Therefore, the identification of high-risk factors of cognitive decline at early stages may be the most effective strategy for the prevention and therapy of dementia.****"*

In the pursuit of such a strategic early intervention to combat cognitive decline, and reverse it before it balloons into full-blown dementia, the research team examined the link between testosterone levels and cognition in approximately 1,300 aging men. Here's what they found:

"Cognitive performance was evaluated by the Consortium to Establish a Registry for Alzheimer's Disease (CERAD) test, Animal Fluency test, and Digit Symbol Substitution Test (DSST)....

In men, higher concentrations of total testosterone were associated with better performance on CERAD test*... Similarly, higher concentrations of free testosterone were associated with better performance on CERAD test...*

Serum testosterone concentrations were inversely associated with cognitive performance in older men*."*

In more digestible terms, the more optimal your testosterone levels are, the more optimally your brain functions.

These findings, again as in the case of mental health, should come as no surprise, given the prevalence of aforementioned androgen receptors in the brain that require testosterone to function at their peak.

It's certainly why I'm not surprised when I see remarkable turnarounds in cognition in my older male patients at my LowTE Florida office following BHRT with bioidentical testosterone.

I have been treating a male attorney patient for years. He says he knows when he needs to come see me because he starts to lose his focus. He says soon after treatment, he feels his brain fog lift and his focus returns. He says he feels confident he is keeping up with the younger attorneys when his hormones are optimized.

Bioidentical Testosterone Increases Energy in Men

Chronic fatigue is one of the most common and debilitating symptoms that men who visit my LowTE Florida office report experiencing.

As a diagnosis, this condition is termed chronic fatigue syndrome (CFS), and often presents in tandem with a reduced sex drive (libido), mood disorders, and a general loss of interest in activities or hobbies that one formerly engaged in with gusto.

Because chronic fatigue is another one of those conditions that have multiple potential underlying causes, clinical expertise, as always, in the diagnostic process is a must. As is often the case, it's common for general medicine practitioners to overlook hormone deficiency as one of the leading causes of chronic fatigue, including in men with low testosterone.

As I have seen firsthand and as the clinical evidence bears out, hormone optimization bioidentical testosterone therapy, for men with low Tis an essential element of maintaining energy levels over time.

Below we have the results of a 2022 study, published in Drugs in Context [9], investigating the fatigue-relieving and energy-enhancing impacts of testosterone replacement therapy for men with low T:

> *"Fatigue is... a concern in [patients with low testosterone], impairing quality of life and well-being...*
>
> *This study compared men with LOH who were already on TRT for >1 year (study group) to men newly diagnosed with LOH who recently started TRT (<1 year; control group) ...*

> ***[Fatigue Severity Score] was significantly higher in the control group compared to TRT >1 year...***
>
> ***Patients treated with TRT >1 year exhibited significantly lower fatigue severity scores...***
>
> *This study further strengthens a growing body of evidence that supports the pivotal role of* ***TRT in individuals with [low testosterone]*** *by adding evidence that it* ***improves fatigue****."*

Clinical data is excellent, but of course the personal patient experience trumps all. Real-world results are what matter to my patients and me.

Check out the testimonials from my male patients, coming up, for true firsthand accounts of rebounding energy levels following BHRT with bioidentical testosterone.

Bioidentical Testosterone Shreds Fat in Men

If you struggle with excess body fat, you're most definitely not alone. An estimated two-thirds of all American adults are either overweight or obese.

This devastating situation is primarily the consequence of a combination of poor diet, lack of exercise, and hormone imbalance.

Highly related to the revved-up metabolism and increased energy levels conferred by bioidentical testosterone is the absolute blowtorch it takes to adipose tissue, known in common parlance as body fat.

The body composition transformations I witness in my male patients at my LowTE Florida office is nothing short of incredible, particularly when combined with optimized diets and exercise.

Consider this glowing endorsement of the practice from the respected medical journal Current Opinion in Endocrinology, Diabetes and Obesity [10], lauding testosterone replacement therapy as "novel" and "timely" for treating obesity in men with low T:

> *"Testosterone therapy in obese men with testosterone deficiency represents a novel and a timely therapeutic strategy for managing obesity in men with testosterone deficiency...*
>
> ***Long-term testosterone therapy in men with testosterone deficiency produces significant and sustained weight loss**, marked reduction in waist circumference and BMI and improvement in body composition. Further, testosterone therapy ameliorates components of the metabolic syndrome...*
>
> *The implication of testosterone therapy in management of obesity in men with testosterone deficiency is of paramount clinical significance, as **it produces sustained weight loss without recidivism. On the contrary, alternative therapeutic approaches other than bariatric surgery failed to produce significant and sustained outcome and exhibit a high rate of recidivism**."*

What that last paragraph means, translated from medical jargon into plain English, is that weight-loss surgery and other therapies intended to treat obesity in the long-term a) fail to work as promised and; b) result in "rebound" weight gain (recidivism). In popular culture, this is often called "yo-yo" weight fluctuations.

In other words, the study results indicate that BHRT with bioidentical testosterone, ideally in combination with healthy lifestyle changes (we'll discuss those in detail in a later chapter) is the gold standard for inducing sustainable weight loss in men with low T.

It has been fun to see my male patients that originally come in with their Tommy Bahama shirts untucked hiding what is going on underneath their shirts coming in a year later with a tight T-shirt and showing off their "guns"! Before we initiate treatment, we perform a body composition measure utilizing the InBody® ~~machine~~ analyzer clearly showing fat vs. muscle throughout the body. It is impressive when we repeat that after a year of treatment and it shows a much healthier ratio. Decreased fat and increased muscle. Of course, the patient's lifestyle contributes to these changes. What I have seen is that once we optimize their hormones, they feel more like exercising and making better food choices.

Bioidentical Testosterone Annihilates Dangerous Chronic Inflammation in Men

The medical community is rapidly developing a consensus, for good reason, that chronic inflammation is the single largest underlying trigger of chronic disease.

Chronic health conditions tied to chronic, untreated inflammation include everything, according to Nature Medicine [11], from cancer to heart disease to autoimmune conditions like rheumatoid arthritis and lupus to neurodegenerative diseases like Alzheimer's, which together affect hundreds of millions of Americans.

Furthermore, the public health burden of chronic inflammation is increasing at an alarming rate with no obvious end in sight.

BHRT with bioidentical testosterone to the rescue?

Let's examine the chronic inflammation-ameliorating effects of bioidentical testosterone as reported via the Journal of Clinical Medicine [12]:

> *"**The benefits of testosterone therapy in ameliorating or attenuating the symptoms of several chronic inflammatory diseases have been reported.** An example of the benefits of testosterone therapy are the improvements noted in patients with Crohn's disease. Crohn's disease patients received standard treatment (without testosterone), apparently without benefits other than maintaining the disease under control during active flare up phases. However, **testosterone therapy not only improved autoimmune disease symptoms in this condition, but also provided added benefits such as improved sexual function, improved body composition, etc.** An increase in muscle mass may*

be the most important benefit in debilitating diseases such as Crohn's and COPD."

There you have it.

The proof is in the pudding: I've seen dramatic health turnarounds in my male patients battling a multitude of conditions associated with chronic inflammation who receive BHRT with bioidentical testosterone at my LowTE Florida office.

Bioidentical Testosterone Spurs Muscle Growth in Men

The progressive loss of muscle mass commonly seen in the aging process, called "sarcopenia," is a well-documented downstream effect of age-related loss of testosterone.

This is logical cause-and-effect, as testosterone is one of the main anabolic (muscle-building) hormones. Without enough of it, muscle is not built or maintained.

Many of my male patients, who have previously been unable to achieve their dream physiques and strength levels, even with intensive dietary changes and regular anabolic exercise like weightlifting, develop substantial new musculature following BHRT with bioidentical testosterone. Without an optimal testosterone level, it is virtually impossible to build muscle. You can tone and keep what you have, but if you want to build muscles, testosterone optimization is critical.

Via the Journal of Clinical Endocrinology and Metabolism [13]:

"Testosterone replacement in hypogonadism has long been known to promote nitrogen retention and increase body density...

Muscle mass was estimated both by excretion of creatinine on a meat-free diet and from appendicular mass measured using dual energy X-ray absorptiometry. Muscle protein synthesis was assessed by measuring the increment of leucine in mixed muscle protein and myosin heavy chain during a continuous infusion of L-leucine.

In all subjects there was an increase in fat-free mass *and a* ***decrease in fat mass****.* ***Muscle mass also increased in everybody*** *such that* ***65% of the increase in fat-free mass could be attributed to accretion of muscle****. The accumulation of muscle was associated with a[n] increase in the fractional synthesis rate of mixed skeletal muscle proteins and a trend toward a similar increase in the fractional synthesis rate of myosin heavy chain. We conclude that* ***testosterone replacement in hypogonadal men enhanced skeletal muscle mass by stimulating the muscle protein synthesis rate****."*

Greater lean muscle mass, along with decreased body fat, is the most noticeable visible transformation that the men receiving bioidentical testosterone therapy at my LowTE Florida exhibit.

And, believe me, their wives and everyone else in their lives take notice.

Bioidentical Testosterone Increases Sex Drive and Hardens Erections in Men

If you switch on the television at any given time, night or day and I don't recommend you do so too often, for your health's sake almost without fail, you're sure to encounter one or more commercials advertising pharmaceutical products called phosphodiesterase-5 (PDE5) inhibitors, sold under the brand names Viagra, Cialis, and Levitra in the United States.

These drugs are designed to facilitate harder, longer-lasting erections in men, particularly older men.

But, while they do have clinical utility for this purpose in many cases, especially in patients with cardiovascular issues, they do not address one fundamental, underlying cause of erectile dysfunction (ED): low testosterone.

From Reviews in Endocrine and Metabolic Disorders [14]:

> *"The specific contribution of low T to sexual function impairment in aging men has still not been completely clarified...*
>
> *Testosterone (T) is a well-recognized crucial factor in regulating male sexual response acting either at a central or peripheral level...*
>
> *The European Male Aging Study (EMAS), a population-based survey performed on more than 3400 men recruited from eight European centers, clearly showed that* ***sexual symptoms—particularly ED, decreased frequency of morning erections and of sexual thoughts—are the most sensitive and specific symptoms in identifying patients with [low testosterone]*** *...*
>
> *Low T is, in fact, often associated with reduced libido, ED, reduced spontaneous erection and delayed ejaculation...*
>
> *Reduced sexual desire is the most important correlate of male hypogonadism."*

Given that sexual dysfunction is the most specific indicator of low T, if you are experiencing any of the symptoms enumerated above and haven't had your testosterone measured, you're missing out on possibly the most efficient (not to mention cost-effective) remedy available.

Stronger erections and a renewed interest in sex are among the most immediately noticeable results of the BHRT with bioidentical testosterone for the male patients visiting my LowTE Florida office. .

Here is the summary of the findings of a comprehensive literature review regarding testosterone therapy to treat issues with sex drive and performance, published in Current Opinion in Urology [15]:

> *"Recent studies have elucidated the role testosterone therapy (TTh) can play in men with low testosterone levels. The aim of this review is to provide an overview of these findings and the utility of TTh.* ***We specifically examine the role of TTh on erectile function, coadministration with phosphodiesterase type 5 inhibitors, and libido****...*
>
> *The available literature supports* ***a role for TTh in men with low testosterone levels, erectile dysfunction, and low libido, with symptomatic improvement in these men****."*

Many of my male patients have reported that their testosterone pellets have increased their libido and helped with ED—giving them a firmer erection that lasts longer. They are very happy.

Bioidentical Testosterone Enhances Immune System Function in Men

If COVID-19 imparted one lesson worth absorbing and applying to our approach to healthcare, it's that we can never be prepared enough immunity-wise to handle what life throws at us.

The environment is absolutely crawling with various pathogenic viruses, bacteria, and fungi, each and every one of these tiny microbes are waiting to take us out—with new ones evolving or potentially artificially created/enhanced through "gain-of-function" scientific research all the time.

If you've ever seen a decomposing body of an animal consumed by bacteria, you understand that entropy is the law of nature: the continual process of creation and destruction.

It's the job of our immune systems, then, to neutralize these environmental threats and keep us healthy. And the good news is that, when we nourish our bodies with the right nutrition, lifestyle practices, and, when necessary, therapeutic intervention, these small but mighty immune systems of ours work extremely well to that end.

It's only when things go wrong with our immune systems that we get sick.

One such thing that can go wrong, and unfortunately often does in older men, is low T.

As with most issues related to hormones, the key word at play is *balance*. In the context of immunity, testosterone and estrogen exert what we might describe as a yin-yang effect; testosterone generally has immune-suppressing effects while estrogen has immune-stimulating effects.

This is why, for example, men (who have higher testosterone levels) tend to be slightly more vulnerable to viral infection while women (who have higher estrogen levels) experience higher rates of autoimmune conditions, in which the immune system is inappropriately overactive and attacks healthy tissue.

What we want is *appropriate*, targeted immune activity to fight off infections without overstimulating the immune system, which can trigger excessive and chronic inflammation, among other undesirable effects (we have previously discussed the serious health threat posed by unchecked inflammation).

Achieving healthy hormone levels, including optimizing testosterone levels, helps us manifest that balance.

In that vein, let's survey the findings of a 2021 study examining the relationship between testosterone levels in men and COVID-19 outcomes, from the Journal of Sexual Medicine [16]:

> *"As SARS-CoV-2 continues to spread, it remains unclear why men disproportionately display higher rates of infection and mortality. While there is no direct evidence that testosterone is directly responsible for the increased susceptibility in men, there is a potential role of testosterone driving ACE-2 and TMPRSS2 to permit viral entry and fusion.* ***The body's inflammatory response is the recognized culprit in those with adverse outcomes****. While testosterone may enhance SARS-CoV-2 viral entry and fusion,* ***it appears that testosterone is protective against immune dysregulation****. Accordingly,* ***men with low testosterone may be more likely to respond with a dangerous inflammatory response***

> ***to the virus and may therefore benefit from testosterone replacement thera****py. Further studies are needed to illuminate the applicability of testosterone replacement therapy in men with SARS-CoV-2."*

Translating into laymen's terms, what this study shows is that the negative outcomes of COVID-19 infection (severe illness or death) are not the result of the viral infection *per se*, but rather the immune system's inflammatory response to it. This overactive immune response includes the dreaded "cytokine storm," which you may have heard of, and which unfortunately claimed many lives during the pandemic.

What the study concludes is that testosterone positively modulates the inflammatory response, thereby limiting negative health outcomes from COVID-19 in men with healthy T counts.

It's no exaggeration, therefore, to say that, if you come down with COVID-19 (or any other viral or bacterial infection), it's possible that your testosterone levels could mean the difference between life and death.

Again, what we aim for is *balance*. If testosterone levels in ratio to estrogen are too high (for example, as seen in steroid abuse), immune system function might be impaired. On the other hand, in testosterone-deficient men, low testosterone can trigger a host of immune system pathologies, including potentially deadly inflammation.

At my LowTE Florida office, we leave nothing to guesswork. I routinely monitor my patients' T levels throughout the process of BHRT with bioidentical testosterone, adjusting dosing as necessary, to get them into that sweet spot for optimal immune system function.

Bioidentical Testosterone Promotes Healthy Sleep in Men

Healthy sleep (7-9 hours of interrupted slumber), along with diet and exercise, is one of the cornerstones of anti-aging health.

(Some individuals, which the medical community sometimes terms "super-sleepers," can function well on fewer hours of sleep, but these are the exceptions to the rule. I advise all my patients to strive for 7-9 hours of quality sleep—easier said than done in our busy world, I know, but nonetheless advice worth heeding.)

Sleep is critical because it's when all the body's ongoing repair work occurs, when your body gets a reprieve from the go-go-go pressures of waking life to reset to baseline and awaken prepared to take on the next day.

Unfortunately, most of us don't get enough sleep, either in terms of quantity (the hours we sleep) or quality (the restfulness of our sleep).

Sleep and testosterone levels in men represent a bit of a catch-22: poor sleep can lower testosterone levels, and low testosterone levels can worsen sleep in a negative health spiral.

BHRT with bioidentical testosterone pellets can dig you out of the hole and restore your sleep so that you can awaken each day rejuvenated and eager to take on what life throws at you.

From the Asian Journal of Andrology [17]:

> *"Experimental data suggest that testosterone may modulate individual vulnerability to subjective symptoms of sleep restriction. Low testosterone may affect overall* ***sleep quality*** *which* ***is improved by replacement doses [of testosterone]****."*

Improved sleep quantity and quality is one of the major benefits that my patients experience after receiving BHRT with bioidentical testosterone, which usually becomes apparent within a few weeks of starting therapy.

And, when your sleep improves, so does literally every other aspect of health we have touched on here.

Bioidentical Testosterone Effectively Treats PTSD in Men

PTSD, or post-traumatic stress disorder, can and does affect men of all ages and occupations, although it is most often associated with the traumas experienced by war veterans.

In addition to combat as a cause, PTSD can be triggered by:

- Unresolved childhood trauma
- Physical trauma like car accidents
- Sexual/physical assault

The symptoms of PTSD can be wide-ranging and include:

- Avoiding places, people, or objects associated with the source of the trauma
- Intrusive, recurring thoughts pertaining to the source of the trauma
- Flashbacks
- Nightmares
- Hopelessness
- Suicidality
- Feelings of detachment

...among many more.

PTSD is far more common than you might believe. Consider these statistics by way of the United States Department of Veterans Affairs (VA) [18]:

> *"About **6 out of every 100 people** (or 6% of the U.S. population) **will have PTSD at some point in their lives**... About 5 out of every 100 adults (or 5%) in the U.S. has PTSD in any given year. In 2020, about 13 million Americans had PTSD."*

So, if you're experiencing any of the symptoms of PTSD, know that there are millions of other men out there going through the same thing.

Psychologists, and health practitioners more broadly, still have a lot to learn about how and why PTSD manifests—and how to effectively treat it.

But we've come a long way in our understanding in the last few decades since PTSD was first recognized as a legitimate condition in 1980 in the Diagnostic and Statistical Manual of Mental Disorders (the so-called "Bible" of psychiatry).

And, you'll not be surprised to learn, after having read this far all about the crucial role that hormones play in overall health, that, for men, testosterone is implicated in the occurrence and severity of PTSD.

Here we have an exciting, relatively new study from 2023 examining the link between sex hormones and PTSD, via Brain Sciences [19]:

> *"**Stress exposure downregulates testosterone** and estradiol receptors in the hippocampus. Exogenous **testosterone administration after exposure to trauma can decrease stress responses**. Testosterone is converted to dihydrotestosterone (DHT) and estradiol, acting on androgen and estradiol receptors. **Testosterone** induces its effect via genomic and non-genomic pathways and exerts **anxiolytic* and anti-depressant effects by these receptors**...*
>
> *Testosterone exerts anxiolytic and antidepressant effects via interaction with CRH receptors and androgen receptors. **Gender is also a significant risk factor for developing PTSD, with women being more susceptible to PTSD following a traumatic event**."*

(*"Anxiolytic" is a clinical term that means "anti-anxiety.")

In summary, the more testosterone a man has, the lesser the stress response to stress-inducing triggers seen in PTSD.

Psychotherapy, cognitive-behavioral therapy, and other treatments may still be required to treat PTSD, depending on the case, but the evidence is clear that BHRT with bioidentical testosterone has a role to play in the healing process in men who have low T.

Bioidentical Testosterone Enhances Overall Quality of Life for Men

As I mentioned in a previous chapter, quality of life (QoL) is a critical metric used by clinicians to quantify overall physical, psychological, and emotional well-being.

A wealth of clinical findings shows that, for men with low testosterone, BHRT with bioidentical testosterone can **substantially** improve quality of life.

For instance, below is the verdict on quality of life and optimized testosterone levels via the medical journal The Aging Male [20]:

> *"As the worldwide population ages, the emphasis on having a reasonable quality of life in old-age is increasing. In men,* ***age-associated testosterone decline is one of the major factors that reduce quality of life****. In patients and the physicians treating them, decreased energy levels and impairments to sex-life are perceived as the most important effects of hypogonadism…*
>
> ***Testosterone can improve the quality of life significantly*** *(to the same level as men with normal testosterone levels)* ***and the more severe the symptoms before treatment, the greater the benefits of testosterone replacement****."*

Furthermore, let's take a brief look at a meta-analysis of several clinical studies looking at the beneficial impact of testosterone therapy on quality of life in men with low T, by way of Andrologia [21]:

> *"Five randomized controlled trials [including] 1,212 patients were included. Fixed-effect model was used to calculate the weighted mean difference of score of Aging Males' Symptom rating scale. Our result reveals that* ***testosterone replacement therapy improves patients' health-related quality of life****."*

TRT Success Stories for Men at LowTE Florida

As I mentioned earlier, no secondhand accounts or scientific research papers trump experiencing the benefits of TRT firsthand.

All the clinical proof is golden—which is why I include so much of it here for you to absorb—but it's the undeniable personal transformation stories that I enjoy sharing most because they demonstrate real-world benefits of this remarkable therapy.

Here's the gracious recollection of the experience of my patient Chris C., via Google Review:

> *"This place is amazing. Carolyn and her team did an amazing job of explaining everything that was going on with my body and suggesting the best course of treatment. They are very warm, attentive, and caring. I felt no pressure at all. I opted for the pellets and three months later, I couldn't be happier with the results and with how I have regained my life and my health. When I first contacted them, I was shocked, confused, and I felt very alone.* ***My primary doctor wasn't on board with hormone replacement therapy and he just expected me to live with low [testosterone] at a relatively young age. LowTE Florida was a blessing. I would give them 10 stars if I could.****"*

Let me tell you something: I hear slightly different variations of this same story *all the time* from patients. They are suffering from hormone deficiencies but either don't receive the hormone therapy that would benefit them so greatly or they don't ever get an accurate diagnosis at all until they come to me.

And, once they *do* get an accurate diagnosis and we get them on the road to success via BHRT, their health and lives turn around in remarkable fashion.

Also, by way of Google Reviews, my patient James L. summarizes his experience with me at LowTE Florida:

"This is by far the best run place I have ever been to. The staff are very professional, knowledgeable, and responsive. What a difference from any other place in South Florida. Even little things like taking care of your annual bloodwork saving you a special trip to the lab is a plus! Carloyn and her staff are top notch. I wish all places were run this well."

"Love this office and Staff. Wonderful people, amazing service and great results from the pellet and supplement regiment. Highly Recommend!" adds John B. via Yelp.

Scores of additional reviews—overwhelmingly glowing—are widely available, including on my website (LowTEFlorida.com), Yelp, Facebook, Google, and more.

Testosterone and the prostate

For over eighty years there has been a fear that testosterone therapy will cause new prostate cancer to arise or hidden ones to grow. However, there has been no scientific studies to back up this assumption. I have followed the teachings of Dr. Abraham Morgentaler from Harvard Medical School for years. He has devoted his life studies to testosterone and prostate cancer. He is very supportive of testosterone therapy for men. In his book ***Testosterone for Life,*** he writes

"I believe the best summary about the risk of prostate cancer from T therapy, based on published evidence at the time this book is written, is as follows:

- Low blood levels of testosterone do not protect against prostate cancer and, indeed, may increase the risk.
- High blood levels of testosterone do not increase the risk of prostate cancer.
- Treatment with testosterone does not increase the risk of prostate cancer, even among men who are already at high risk for it."

More and more physicians are learning that testosterone therapy is not a true risk for prostate cancer and are finding testosterone is supportive for a healthy prostate. The thought of a high testosterone causing prostate cancer just has never made sense to me. Men's testosterone is at it's highest when they are in their late teens and early twenties. How many of those guys have prostate cancer? I would believe the number is close to zero.

I have several patients that have had prostate cancer and a prostatectomy (complete removal of the prostate. One their PSA is zero – we are good to go ahead with testosterone treatment. Of course, I like to get their doctors blessing – but we have not seen any problems with these patients. Many comment how much better they feel with the testosterone therapy.

References

[1] United States Institute of Medicine. (2004). Testosterone and Aging: Clinical Research Directions. United States Institute of Medicine. https://www.ncbi.nlm.nih.gov/books/NBK216164/

[2] Tokish, J., DeRosa, D. (2014). Pharmacologic Approaches to the Aging Athlete. Sports Health. https://www.ncbi.nlm.nih.gov/pmc/articles/PMC3874227/

[3] Yeap, B., Marriot, R. (2024). Associations of Testosterone and Related Hormones With All-Cause and Cardiovascular Mortality and Incident Cardiovascular Disease in Men. Annals of Internal Medicine. https://www.acpjournals.org/doi/10.7326/M23-2781

[4] Urology Care Foundation. (n.d.) What Is Low Testosterone? https://www.urologyhealth.org/urology-a-z/l/low-testosterone

[5] Rubin, R. (2024). The Most Exciting Time for Testosterone. Medscape. https://www.medscape.com/viewarticle/999636?form=fpf

[6] Sharma, R., Oni, O., et al. (2015). Normalization of testosterone level is associated with reduced incidence of myocardial infarction and mortality in men. European Heart Journal. https://academic.oup.com/eurheartj/article/36/40/2706/2293361

[7] Walther, A., Breidenstein, J., et al. (2018). Association of Testosterone Treatment With Alleviation of Depressive Symptoms in Men: A Systematic Review and Meta-analysis. Journal of the American Medical Association. https://pubmed.ncbi.nlm.nih.gov/30427999/

[8] Dong, X., Jiang, H., et al. (2021). Low Serum Testosterone Concentrations Are Associated With Poor Cognitive Performance in Older Men but Not Women. Frontiers in Aging Neuroscience. https://www.frontiersin.org/articles/10.3389/fnagi.2021.712237/full

[9] de Almeida Ferreira, M. and Alexandre Mendonça, J. (2022). Drugs in Context. https://www.ncbi.nlm.nih.gov/pmc/articles/PMC8823386/

[10] Traish, A. (2014). Testosterone and weight loss: the evidence. Current Opinion in Endocrinology, Diabetes and Obesity. https://pubmed.ncbi.nlm.nih.gov/25105998/

[11] Furman, D., Campisi, J., et al. (2019). Chronic inflammation in the etiology of disease across the life span. Nature Medicine. https://www.ncbi.nlm.nih.gov/pmc/articles/PMC7147972/

[12] Traish, A., Bolanos, A., et al. (2018). Do Androgens Modulate the Pathophysiological Pathways of Inflammation? Appraising the Contemporary Evidence. Journal of Clinical Medicine. https://www.ncbi.nlm.nih.gov/pmc/articles/PMC6306858

[13] Brodsky, I., Balagopal, P., et al. (1996). Effects of testosterone replacement on muscle mass and muscle protein synthesis in hypogonadal men--a clinical research center study. The Journal of Clinical Endocrinology and Metabolism. https://pubmed.ncbi.nlm.nih.gov/8855787/

[14] Corona, G. and Maggi, M. (2022). The role of testosterone in male sexual function. Reviews in Endocrine and Metabolic Disorders. https://www.ncbi.nlm.nih.gov/pmc/articles/PMC9789013/

[15] Rizk, P., Kohn, T. (2017). Testosterone Therapy Improves Erectile Function and Libido in Hypogonadal Men. Current Opinion in Urology. https://www.ncbi.nlm.nih.gov/pmc/articles/PMC5649360/

[16] Auerbach, J. and Khera, M. (2021). Testosterone's Role in COVID-19. The Journal of Sexual Medicine. https://www.ncbi.nlm.nih.gov/pmc/articles/PMC7972673/

[17] Wittert, G. (2014). The relationship between sleep disorders and testosterone in men. Asian Journal of Andrology. https://www.ncbi.nlm.nih.gov/pmc/articles/PMC3955336/

[18] United States Department of Veterans Affairs. (n.d.) How Common Is PTSD in Adults? United States Department of Veterans Affairs. https://www.ptsd.va.gov/understand/common/common_adults.asp

[19] Raise, Abdullahi, P., Meamar, M., et al. (2023). Hypothalamus and Post-Traumatic Stress Disorder: A Review. Brain Sciences. https://www.ncbi.nlm.nih.gov/pmc/articles/PMC10377115/

[20] Moncada, I. (2006). Testosterone and men's quality of life. The Aging Male. https://pubmed.ncbi.nlm.nih.gov/17178553/

[21] Nian, Y., Ding, M. (2017). Testosterone replacement therapy improves health-related quality of life for patients with late-onset hypogonadism: a meta-analysis of randomized controlled trials. Andrologia. https://pubmed.ncbi.nlm.nih.gov/27389320/

[22] Morgentaler, A. (2009). Testosterone for Life. McGraw Hill.

Chapter VIII

What is Pellet Therapy and Why is it the Best Method for Hormone Optimization?

The delivery methods of bioidentical hormones, thanks to advances in the science behind this exciting form of therapy, have evolved over the years.

The vehicle I prefer, that I predominately use in my practice at LowTE Florida, is the small but mighty bioidentical hormone "pellet," for reasons I'll explain here.

Good things, as the saying goes, come in small packages. Hormone pellets owe their name to their small size, implanted subcutaneously (the medical term for "under the skin") in a quick out-patient procedure in my office.

Here are a few of the advantages provided by using pellets for BHRT over other methods:

- Pellets require no effort or upkeep on the part of the patient. In fact, as many of my patients tell me, you will likely forget you have one implanted until you start to notice the improvements
- Pellets are discreet; no one in your family or extended social circle will know you are using one, unless you tell them
- Pellets provide a continuous, steady supply of hormones
- Pellets are perfect for patients who don't like needles or taking pills every day

Bioidentical hormone pellets (roughly the size of a Tic-Tac® for reference) are the gold standard of hormone therapy, as they enable a consistent, steady supply of all-natural hormones—testosterone and estradiol (for women)—into the bloodstream where it then has access to nourish all the tissues and organs that need it.

Aside from the constant infusion of hormones into the bloodstream, the other major upside of pellets as the delivery mechanism for BHRT is their convenience: once it's in, you never have to think about it again until your next office visit—no fretting about dosing, no needles, no remembering to take your pills, no nighttime rituals with creams.

Let's run down the essential process of BHRT using bioidentical hormone pellets that I utilize with my patients in my LowTE Florida office, which can be performed easily in just a few minutes:

- Apply local anesthesia (a numbing agent) to the upper buttocks area (this is the only part you may feel—takes about 5 seconds)
- Finesse the pellet under the skin with surgical precision utilizing an instrument to place it a few inches away from the small (less than a quarter inch) incision
- The patient is out the door and back to their life
- The pellet will remain intact, working its science-backed magic while it dissolves over a period of 3-6 months (men generally require new pellet insertions every 4-6 months while women require new pellet insertions every 3-5 months)
- We want you to have your hormone levels tested with a blood test 4-6 weeks after the first pellet insertion procedure. We then review the original symptom list and evaluate the lab results. If you still have symptoms, and the lab test indicates that you could benefit from more, we have you come in for a "boost"—meaning more pellets to get you to the level that gives you the desired benefits of the therapy at no charge. I am a bit conservative with my first dosing—I just want you to get to the "feel good" levels safely and comfortably
- Return for an evaluation of progress, with dose adjustments as needed, and insertion of new pellets. In my practice, I have five different doses of bioidentical testosterone and five different doses of bioidentical estradiol (the bioidentical form of estrogen) at my disposal. This allows me to adjust the dose each patient receives to match his or her individual needs and goals on an ongoing basis for maximum efficacy

I have supreme confidence in the power of the pellet because I've seen it up close. Not only with my patients, but I have been a satisfied pellet patient for 11+ years! Within a matter of weeks, my patients reliably report noticeable resolution of their symptoms and improvements in their vitality and sense of well-being, including:

- Improved mood/outlook on life
- Restored mental acuity (cognition)
- Increased energy levels
- Reignited sex drive (libido)
- Better sleep quality

...Just to name a few of the most common life-enhancing effects of bioidentical hormone pellets.

Convenience and maximum efficacy never came in such an assuming form. The pellets are the safest delivery system for hormones. We have the highest quality pellets for our patients. One pellet from each batch is tested eight different ways to assure sterility, strength, contents, compactness, etc.

In addition to hormone pellets, in my practice I also utilize (when necessary for logistical reasons or due to patient preference) creams, pills, troches, and shots containing bioidentical testosterone, estrogen, and progesterone. However, in my experience, the pellet treatment is far superior giving a nice consistent delivery of the hormones rather than a roller coaster effect from the other delivery systems. Why would I give you a Volkswagen (other delivery systems) when I can give you a Rolls-Royce (pellets)?

Potential Negatives of BHRT

As with any procedure or treatment there are ***potential*** risks involved. However, at LowTE Florida, you can have the confidence that we do everything in our power for you to have a safe and comfortable experience. You can also have the confidence that if any untoward effects appear, we know how to handle them to get you feeling and looking your best. I am very conservative with dosing – going low and slow in the beginning until we are able to dial in the perfect dose – this helps prevent many of the potential side effects from appearing.

In the case of BHRT pellets, we have seen the minimal side effects are by far outweighed by the life changing results of the therapy. We have a 97% return rate after the first pellet – which tells you that for most people the good outweighs the bad. Going to a reputable hormone expert is key. Proper dosing is key, and the pellet procedure must be done correctly.

For women, what I hear from the patients is they may notice an increase in facial hair and a small percentage report increased acne. Hair thinning and a slightly enlarged clitoris are reported rarely and can be treated. However, adjusting the dose at the next pellet usually resolves these issues. The literature shows no increase in blood pressure, cholesterol or blood sugar.

For men, their sperm count will go down – so if you are planning a pregnancy in the next seven months, it is better to wait until your partner is pregnant before initiating treatment. The other potential side effects are minimal. If the patient doesn't follow the post-procedure rules for the first 7-10 days after the pellet procedure - no swimming, soaking, hot tub or baths and no heavy work outs, you may extrude the pellets after about the first month. You don't want this to happen, so it is imperative that you follow direction. Walking is fine – just for those 7-10 days then you can get back to it. Infections are very rare but easily treated.

It is important that we monitor your labs. In a small percentage of men, we may see an increase in red blood cells (hemoglobin and hematocrit). If we see this, we have a protocol to help correct this and then we can adjust the dose at the next pellet procedure. Also, a small minority of the male patients may have an increase in estradiol. While men need a little estradiol, they don't need a lot. Again, we have a protocol if we see this on the labs four weeks after the pellet. And just as we insist on mammograms for women – we need to see PSA levels for men on a regular basis. Not that the pellets cause changes in these areas – we just want to know that you are healthy and not missing significant health changes.

The potential side effects of bioidentical hormone pellet therapy compared to synthetic hormones are far better. As we covered before, the synthetic (not bioidentical) oral treatment may lead to blood clots, heart attack, stroke and breast cancer. I have not seen in the literature any correlation with bioidentical hormones and clotting changes.

With the pellets the hormones are absorbed directly into your blood stream. They are not time-released, they are cardio released. If your heart rate is higher (with exercise or stress) you may pick up more hormones as your blood passes by the pellets. Which is good - you will have better results with the pellets. Meaning, if you start feeling great and training for a marathon, you may burn through the pellets a little quicker than if you choose to be a couch potato.

Testosterone and estradiol pellets have a strong safety profile (used in the US for over 80 years and they remain to this day the most effective hormone treatment and the safest way to get hormones inside your body.

Chapter IX
Thyroid Disease: The Silent Epidemic

In this section, we're going to take a deep dive into a small, but powerful (and very much under-appreciated) gland located at the base of your neck: the mighty thyroid.

Why do I test for thyroid hormones when patients are coming in for "Bioidentical Hormone Therapy"? Because I learned early on that the symptoms of low thyroid can overlap with low sex hormones. I don't want to fix one thing and have you still not feeling your best.

The thyroid gland sits centered on the lower part of your neck. When it gets inflamed and/or enlarged, you can often feel it as a lump in your throat. An inflamed thyroid, which can happen due to multiple reasons, is a condition called thyroiditis, while an enlarged thyroid gland is called goiter.

The two thyroid hormones, produced by the thyroid's follicular epithelial cells, which are critical for optimal health, are:

- Triiodothyronine (aka T3)
- Tetraiodothyronine (aka T4)

A third hormone implicated strongly in thyroid function, though not technically speaking a thyroid hormone itself, is thyroid-stimulating hormone (TSH), produced in the pituitary gland in the brain.

Without getting too deep into the physiology weeds (I know this isn't a biology lesson), TSH's job in the complex hormone feedback loop is to stimulate the production of T4, which in turn stimulates the synthesis of bioactive T3 by the liver and kidneys, which in turn nourishes every major cell, tissue, and organ in the body.

Together, these thyroid hormones are critical for regulation of:

- body temperature

- mental clarity
- energy
- heart rate
- blood pressure
- metabolism
- hair
- mood

...and much more.

The two major (but not the only) ways that the thyroid can become dysfunctional are:

- **Hyperthyroidism**. This refers to an overactive thyroid, in which too much T3 and T4 are manufactured, resulting in a variety of symptoms like unwanted weight loss, insatiable appetite, insomnia, and goiter.
- **Hypothyroidism**. This refers to an underactive thyroid, in which too little T3 and T4 are manufactured, resulting in thinning hair, unwanted weight gain, chronic fatigue, depression, and joint and muscle pain.

Of the two, *hypo*thyroidism (thyroid deficiency) is more common, especially in women, and even more especially in older ones.

The clinical literature indicates that hypothyroidism occurs with a 4-5 times greater frequency than hyperthyroidism, and this estimated ratio is accurate according to my personal experience treating patients with thyroid issues hands-on at my LowTE Florida practice.

Thyroid problems, in fact, are among the most common hormone issues and are, unfortunately, commonly undiagnosed or misdiagnosed (a common theme, you'll notice, in modern healthcare), leading to increased risk of heart disease and other chronic, potentially fatal health conditions, as explained via the Journal of Clinical Endocrinology & Metabolism [1]:

> *"**Thyroid dysfunction** is one of the leading endocrine disorders. It **represents around 30% to 40% of the patients seen in an***

> ***endocrine practice.*** *The American Association of Clinical Endocrinologists (AACE) estimated that* ***in the United States approximately 13 million people, or 4.78% of the population, have undiagnosed thyroid dysfunction...***
>
> ***Thyroid hormone excess and deficiency are frequently misunderstood and are too often overlooked and misdiagnosed.*** *Morbidity associated with thyroid dysfunction is well known with deleterious consequences in terms of both elevated serum cholesterol levels and increased risk of coronary artery disease and cardiovascular mortality"*

So, how do we, your anti-aging hormone care experts at LowTE Florida, determine if your thyroid is working properly, and, if it's not, what can we do about it?

Let's discuss.

Is Your Thyroid Whacked?

Do you wake up feeling exhausted?

Are your energy levels so cooked at the end of your workday that you just want to sink into the couch and be done?

If so, you're not alone: **fatigue is the number one reason patients come to LowTE Florida**—followed by unwanted weight gain.

Medical News Today [2] recently, in December 2023, reported on shocking findings from the CDC that the number of Americans suffering from clinically significant and mostly undiagnosed chronic fatigue is much, much higher than previously believed:

> *"The Centers for Disease Control and Prevention (CDC) released the results of a survey in which Americans report receiving a diagnosis of myalgic encephalomyelitis/chronic fatigue syndrome (ME/CFS).*

> *According to the survey,* ***over 1.3% of Americans say their doctor told them they have chronic fatigue syndrome****. Based on the current U.S. population of 333 million, 1.3% of* ***that figure equals about 4.3 million Americans****.*
>
> *The* ***CDC's previous estimate*** *for Americans with CFS/ME* ***was 836,000 to 2.5 million people****.*
>
> *The CDC also reports that about 90% of people with the condition have not been diagnosed."*

So, if we take the figure of 4.3 million Americans, and then consider that the CDC reports that number might only represent 10% of Americans who have chronic fatigue syndrome, then extrapolate, we're talking about potentially **north of 40 million Americans impacted by chronic fatigue**!

Connecting the dots here, one of the defining features of hypothyroidism—the clinical term for chronically low thyroid hormone levels, or thyroid deficiency—is chronic fatigue, as explained in research on hormone therapy for chronic fatigue via Biomedicines [3]:

> *"Fatigue is defined as 'a sense of physical tiredness and lack of energy, distinct from sadness or weaknesses. The most recent definitions refer to fatigue as a suboptimal psychophysiological condition caused by exertion; this state causes changes that may reduce mental processing or physical activity.* ***Fatigue*** *is related with alterations in muscle activity, proprioception, and cognitive function, and* ***has been associated with chronic diseases such as hypothyroidism****. It has been reported that* ***up to one-third of patients presenting with fatigue have thyroid disease****, predominantly in women...*

The Many Faces of Thyroid Deficiency

It's by no means just chronic fatigue that's associated with thyroid dysfunction, which, as we mentioned previously, can manifest in numerous ways.

Maybe you are a bit heavier than you used to be—possibly some brain fog? Is your hair thinning?

A sluggish thyroid can lead to multiple signs and symptoms, including:

- Increased body fat
- Chronically low energy levels
- Depressed, lethargic mood
- Thinning hair
- Cognitive fog (lack of mental clarity)
- Reduced sense of overall well-being

Like testosterone and estrogen deficiencies, low thyroid levels are often general and widespread, resulting in frequent misdiagnosis by general medicine practitioners, as the symptoms of impaired thyroid function are mistaken for other chronic conditions and non-hormone experts lack the training and clinical experience to recognize the signs of thyroid deficiency.

The Art and Science of Diagnosing Thyroid Deficiency

If you're suffering from the ravages of untreated hypothyroidism, a simple blood test can prove that it isn't your fault; you are simply not producing as much thyroid hormone as you did a few years back.

Conventional medicine practitioners tend to rely on only one blood test to evaluate the thyroid: thyroid stimulating hormone (TSH).

At LowTE Florida, we dig deeper, checking on the thyroid hormones that are being utilized throughout your body (Free T3 and T4), not just the thyroid stimulating hormone (TSH), which just indicates what is going on between your thyroid gland and your brain.

(For a more fulsome exploration of the thyroid and its related hormones, head over to LowTEFlorida.com and look for my interview with renowned endocrinologist Dr. Gary Pepper, MD.) We treat hypothyroidism similarly.

Treating Thyroid Deficiency Using Bioidentical Hormone Replacement Therapy

If, in fact, the simple combination of blood tests of TSH, FreeT3, Total T4 levels and TPO Antibodies come back indicating a thyroid deficiency, we move on to treatment.

As always at LowTE Florida, we prescribe for the treatment of hypothyroidism not the synthetic thyroid hormone (levothyroxine or Synthroid®) that you would receive at a conventional medical facility but rather bioidentical hormone replacement therapy using **desiccated bioidentical thyroid hormone extract NP Thyroid® or Armour® Thyroid.**

Even mainline medical associations like the American Thyroid Association [4] have come around to recognize the superior therapeutic value of desiccated bioidentical thyroid hormone extract as compared to the synthetic form of T4, levothyroxine, traditionally used in mainline medical institutions:

> *"Levothyroxine is the main thyroid hormone produced by the thyroid gland and the synthetic form is the most common form of thyroid hormone replacement therapy. Prior to the availability of the pure levothyroxine, desiccated animal thyroid extract was the only treatment for hypothyroidism. Today, some individuals prefer desiccated thyroid extract as a more "natural" thyroid hormone. In addition, some* ***patients who continue to have symptoms of hypothyroidism when taking levothyroxine report improvement in these symptoms when switched to desiccated thyroid extract****...*

Although desiccated thyroid extract is not widely used, this study showed that ***many patients preferred this option as compared with levothyroxine.*** *"*

The bottom line is that desiccated bioidentical thyroid extract works more effectively and with fewer side effects compared to levothyroxine, which is why clinical evidence shows that patients respond more favorably than with synthetic levothyroxine.

As opposed to synthetic levothyroxine, which is termed a "monotherapy" as it only elevates T4 levels, desiccated bioidentical thyroid restores both circulating T3 *and* T4 levels for superior results, as detailed via Annals of Internal Medicine [5]:

"Authors have questioned the efficacy of l-thyroxine monotherapy because about 10% to 15% of patients are dissatisfied as a result of residual symptoms of hypothyroidism, *including neurocognitive impairment, and about 15% of patients do not achieve normal serum triiodothyronine levels.*

Studies of several animal models indicate that maintaining normal serum T3 levels is a biological priority. Although the clinical significance of relatively low serum T3 in humans is not well-defined, evidence shows that elevating serum T3 through the administration of both l-thyroxine and l-triiodothyronine has benefited some patients. However, this has not been consistently demonstrated across trials. Novel findings highlight the molecular mechanisms underlying the inability of l-thyroxine monotherapy to universally normalize measures of thyroid hormone signaling, and new evidence may lay the foundation for a role of personalized medicine. Understanding the historical rationale for the trend toward l-thyroxine monotherapy allows us to identify scientific and clinical targets for future trials."

I explain to my patients that are on Synthroid or Levothyroxine that right now they are getting just T4—a storage unit of thyroid that must be converted by your body to T3 before you can use it. Many people are not converting to T3 well—producing a low Free T3 on the labs. Switching to desiccated thyroid is like making a deposit in your savings account (T4) to be used later AND T3 is like your checking account that you can use today. So, you can feel better and your body can function better today.

These findings are not surprising, given that, as we have discussed at great length in a previous chapter, each of the body's hormones exist in careful balance with all the others.

This is as true with the thyroid hormones as it is with the sex hormones; for optimal health, your body requires T3 and T4 not just in sufficient quantities on their own but in proper balance with, and ratio to, one another—a critical nuance that too often goes unappreciated in conventional medicine.

Let me tell you about my personal experience with desiccated thyroid, so that you can better appreciate the difference it's made in my own life, and what it could do for you as well:

When I studied hormone replacement years ago, I was taught thyroid replacement. I tested my free T3 *(on the lab report it is Triiodothyronine (T3) Free)* and it was in the normal range but on the low end (2.3) and the reference range was 2.0-4.4. My goal with treatment in my LowTE clinical practice is to have the free T3 in the upper quartile of the reference range (3.8-4.2).

Once I started on desiccated thyroid, I didn't notice much of a difference in the beginning—I really didn't think I needed it. But one Saturday I found myself feeling sluggish and not thinking as quickly and clearly as I had been. "Maybe I missed my thyroid pill and that will explain these sluggish feelings," I thought.

I had gotten in the habit of always laying out my thyroid pill on a small dish next to the bed the night before so I could take it first thing when I woke up.

So, to investigate, I went to the dish—but found no pill! Then I look at my 125-pound Labrador, Dominic, who is usually a couch potato, and he was all zipped up! He wanted to go in the pool, go for a run, etc., Wow! I wanted what he had! So, I took my thyroid pill and thirty minutes later we were both in the pool having a great time! I have been taking it regularly ever since.

Hashimoto's Thyroiditis

Rounding out our discussion of the thyroid and thyroid hormones, one other test I include on our initial blood panel is **Thyroid Peroxidase Antibodies (TPO)**.

I perform this test for all my LowTE Florida patients because a high level of TPO antibodies is an indication of Hashimoto's thyroiditis, an autoimmune disorder where antibodies damage your thyroid gland and cause inflammation and hypothyroidism.

There are many books on Hashimoto's thyroiditis that dive deep into what triggers it in your body. I keep it simple, informing my patients with "Hashi's" of four steps they can take that can help them live and feel better:

1) Go totally gluten free. People with Hashimoto's thyroiditis donot process food made from wheat as well as those without this autoimmune disease. When they eat wheat, they may feel bloated and experiencing restless sleep, constipation, and low energy. The gluten is causing inflammation in your abdomen. Many experts are also advising patients with Hashimoto's to watch their lactose (dairy) intake as well.

2) Optimize your thyroid with desiccated thyroid.

3) Take a good probiotic (LowTE Probiotic comes in a patented capsule form that opens in the beginning of the small intestine —giving all the good microbiota the best chance at repairing the lining of the intestines). All autoimmune diseases are based

in the gut, so it makes sense to get your intestines as healthy as possible.

4) Iodine supplementation. In review of the literature, the experts on Hashimoto's appeared to be divided on their opinion on supplementation with iodine. I encourage it both because research indicates that as many as two billion people worldwide suffer from iodine deficiency and because many LowTE Florida patients have told me how much better they feel when they add iodine to their supplement regimen.
We have a very specific protocol for starting iodine supplements. If you take too much too quickly, you can feel poorly, including experiencing flu-like symptoms. So, if you are starting LowTE Iodine Plus, please call the office to learn how to comfortably optimize your dose.

Bioidentical Desiccated Thyroid Hormone Extract Success Stories at LowTE Florida

Let's take a brief look at a sampling of my LowTE Florida patients who came to me with (often undiagnosed) hypothyroidism—whose energy levels, mental health, weight loss, and overall quality of life improved dramatically following bioidentical hormone replacement therapy with bioidentical thyroid hormone extract.

My LowTE Florida patient Angela R. reports "incredible" energy gains and "feeling good again" following our treatment of her hypothyroidism:

> *"I was at an all-time low in my life. I had no desire to work out, have sex or do much at all. I felt like my body was shifting into old-age, and I needed to make a change.* ***After I met Carolyn, she found out that my hormone levels were severely low, and that I also have hypothyroid! Carolyn has not only helped to treat me but changed my life!*** *Today, I work out five days a week with excitement, and my energy is incredible. I feel good again!"*

Tracy G., by way of Google Reviews, simply had the following to offer regarding her experience at LowTE Florida:

> *"Love Carolyn and her team! She straightened out my thyroid and I'm feeling MUCH better!"*

These are real-life people who reaped real-life rewards from bioidentical hormone therapy with bioidentical thyroid, even when conventional medicine failed to either accurately diagnose or effectively treat their conditions.

If you believe your thyroid might be "whacked," based on the nonspecific symptoms we've described here (chronic fatigue, unwanted weight gain, hair loss, etc.), give our friendly LowTE Florida staff a call.

We'll do the proper clinical investigative work and, where appropriate, restore your thyroid hormones to healthy levels via proven bioidentical hormone replacement therapy.

References

[1] Madariaga, A., Palacios, S., et al. (2014). The Incidence and Prevalence of Thyroid Dysfunction in Europe: A Meta-Analysis. The Journal of Clinical Endocrinology & Metabolism. https://academic.oup.com/jcem/article/99/3/923/2537300?login=false

[2] Berman, R. (2023). Chronic fatigue syndrome more common than previous estimates, CDC says. Medical News Today. https://www.medicalnewstoday.com/articles/chronic-fatigue-syndrome-higher-than-previous-estimates-cdc-survey

[3] Ruíz-Pacheco, M., Hernandez, R., et al. (2023). Severity of Fatigue and Its Relationship with TSH before and after Levothyroxine Replacement Therapy in Patients with Primary Hypothyroidism. Biomedicines. https://www.ncbi.nlm.nih.gov/pmc/articles/PMC10045891/

[4] American Thyroid Association. (2013). Desiccated thyroid extract vs Levothyroxine in the treatment of hypothyroidism. American Thyroid Association. https://www.thyroid.org/patient-thyroid-information/ct-for-patients/vol-6-issue-8/vol-6-issue-8-p-3/

[5] McAninch, E. and Bianco, A. (2016). The History and Future of Treatment of Hypothyroidism. Annals of Internal Medicine. https://www.ncbi.nlm.nih.gov/pmc/articles/PMC4980994/

Chapter X
The Vital Role of Targeted, Strategic Supplementation for Your Best Health

As we'll discuss in the next chapter, cleaning up your diet, followed by getting regular exercise and achieving optimal sleep, is arguably the single most important basic step you can take to ensure a long, healthy, active life.

Diet is still king, but the reality is that, especially as we age, sourcing all of the nutritional sustenance we need from food alone is not possible for most people in our toxic modern world, especially given the phenomenon of soil depletion—a term referencing the removal of crucial vitamins and minerals from the soil that food is grown in due to numerous causes, including industrial farming techniques.

To understand the devastating effects of soil depletion on human nutrition, let's turn to Scientific American [1]:

> *"**Fruits and vegetables grown decades ago were much richer in vitamins and minerals than the varieties most of us get today**. The main culprit in this disturbing nutritional trend is soil depletion: Modern intensive agricultural methods have stripped increasing amounts of nutrients from the soil in which the food we eat grows. Sadly, each successive generation of fast-growing, pest-resistant carrot is truly less good for you than the one before...*
>
> ***A Kushi Institute analysis of nutrient data from 1975 to 1997 found that average calcium levels in 12 fresh vegetables dropped 27 percent; iron levels 37 percent; vitamin A levels 21 percent, and vitamin C levels 30 percent**. A similar study of British nutrient data from 1930 to 1980, published in the British Food Journal, found that in 20 vegetables the average calcium content had*

declined 19 percent; iron 22 percent; and potassium 14 percent. Yet another study concluded ***that one would have to eat eight oranges today to derive the same amount of Vitamin A as our grandparents would have gotten from one.****"*

YIKES!

The saving grace (your protection against the negative effects of soil depletion) is that, through targeted, personalized supplementation regimens that I develop with each of my patients, we can make up for many nutritional deficiencies in your diet via top-rated, purity-tested, patented LowTE Florida supplements.

Coming up, we'll run down a few of the most effective LowTE Florida supplements I use for patients in my clinical practice, each one an excellent complement to a healthy diet and hormone optimization that you stand to benefit from in your own life, particularly as you advance in age.

Bear in mind that each of these industry-leading supplements is uniquely formulated and patented by LowTE Florida, meaning you can only get them through my office, website, or Amazon. Our expert team of researchers go to great lengths developing and testing these products to ensure they deliver the promised results—so accept no substitutes!

When developing my proprietary supplements, in collaboration with industry-leading partners, I use three basic metrics, my north stars to supplement creation:

1. **Does this particular compound work as promised**? What does the totality of the research (not just one or two cherry-picked studies) say about its therapeutic benefits?
2. **Is the dosage correct** to achieve the intended results? What does the research say about the optimal dose? Is it enough to achieve the intended results but not so much as to cause adverse effects?

3. **Is the supplement, as formulated, bioavailable**? The term "bioavailability" refers to the body's ability to process, absorb, and distribute a given medicinal compound.
   It doesn't matter how great any particular supplement is if it doesn't get into the cells, tissues, and organs that it's intended to.
   In my opinion, this is where supplements often go wrong. Your standard grocery store multivitamin, for instance, is mostly a waste of money because many of the ingredients are not absorbed by the gut and are simply passed through the urine or feces.
   My priority, therefore, is to make any necessary modifications to my LowTE Florida products to ensure maximum bioavailability so the medicinal compounds get into the cells and tissues where they belong.

I send out my supplement line regularly to an outside testing laboratory to assure that what is on the label is actually in the capsule—and nothing more. Years ago, I sold a supplement provided by a well- known company. I learned that the outside lab testing showed it was inert! No active ingredients! That is what spurred me on to develop my LowTE Florida line of nutritional supplements that I could have control over.

For further information, all of our products have their own respective pages at my website, https://lowteflorida.com/store, complete with comprehensive product details, pricing information (including discount codes), details regarding our money-back satisfaction guarantee, as well as links to relevant published research, and more.

LowTE Florida DIM

Diindolylmethane, often abbreviated as simply DIM, is a powerful modulator of sex hormone levels for men and women alike, an adjunct therapy I use with all my bioidentical hormone replacement therapy patients because of its powerful therapeutic action on the hormone system. I recommend LowTE Florida DIM supplement to both my male and female patients on BHRT.

For a quick biochemistry lesson on the origins of DIM, if you have taken any kind of dive into the fascinating world of nutrition, then you might be familiar with a potent medicinal compound naturally occurring in cruciferous vegetables (the class of veggies that includes spinach, broccoli, cauliflower, etc.) called indole-3-carbinol (I3C), a compounded noted for its prophylactic effects on cancer as well as its heart health-promoting and obesity-fighting properties.

Let's take a page out of the clinical literature published in Advances in Experimental Medicine and Biology [2]:

> ***"Indole-3-carbinol (I3C),*** *a common phytochemical in cruciferous vegetables,* ***and its condensation product, 3,3'-diindolylmethane (DIM) exert several biological activities on cellular and molecular levels,*** *which contribute to their well-recognized chemoprevention potential. Initially, these compounds were classified as blocking agents that increase drug-metabolizing enzyme activity. Now it is widely accepted that* ***I3C and DIM affect multiple signaling pathways and target molecules controlling cell division, apoptosis, or angiogenesis deregulated in cancer cells.*** *Although most of the current data support the role of I3C and DIM in prevention of hormone-dependent cancers, it seems that* ***their application in prevention of the other cancer as well as cardiovascular disease, obesity, and diabetes reduction is also possible.*** *This chapter summarizes the current experimental data on the I3C and DIM activity and the results of clinical studies indicating their role in prevention of chronic diseases."*

As explained above, DIM is the bioactive breakdown of indole-3-carbinol, so it's the ultimate form of the "good stuff" in cruciferous veggies that works therapeutically on the cells and tissues that benefit.

While it's possible to source a modest amount of DIM from the diet through the metabolic mechanisms explained above, what my DIM supplement does is pack a concentrated form of the compound into a single pill, far beyond what you would obtain from your average kale salad, which exponentially maximizes its therapeutic effectiveness.

In addition to protecting the heart, preventing diabetes, and combatting cancer, DIM also powerfully modulates sex hormone ratios to correct numerous issues in both men and women caused by hormone imbalance, including acne, prostate enlargement in men, hot flashes in women experiencing menopause, and more.

I know my exclusive DIM supplement works as promised—and better than competing brands—because my LowTE Florida patients give me firsthand raving feedback regularly during our visits and in posted reviews:

> "I have never felt better since I started taking DIM! Taking it for years and would highly recommend it," offers LowTE Florida patient David S.
>
> "I had an allergic reaction to [a different DIM supplement from another company] ... My sister recommended I try her DIM supplement—LowTE Florida, which she uses. I have been taking the LowTE Florida DIM for four days now without any allergic reaction. I think this is a much safer DIM supplement for me to take," writes patient Karen F. "Additionally, I had a question about where the product was sourced and manufactured and the owner of LowTE Florida (Carolyn Z.) called me personally to discuss the measures they take to ensure the integrity of the supplement." "I am very pleased with the product and customer service at LowTE Florida," she added.

LowTE Florida Vitamin D (ADK5/ADK 10)

Our proprietary LowTE Florida ADK 5 & 10 supplements synergistically blends the following three highly bioavailable forms of:

- Vitamin D (as cholecalciferol)
- Vitamin A (as retinyl palmitate)

- Vitamin K (as menaquinone-7, or MK-7)

If there were just one nutrient deficiency that I would encourage anyone visiting my LowTE Florida office to get tested for, it's your vitamin D status, for several reasons that I'll explain briefly here.

(As a side note, the term "vitamin D" is a bit of a misnomer, as it is more accurately classified physiologically as a steroid hormone, more similar in its structure and mechanism of action to testosterone and estrogen than, for example, vitamin A or C. But we'll continue to refer to it as "vitamin D" because that's the term everyone is already familiar with.)

The first reason I recommend everyone monitor their vitamin D levels is that we in the medical and research community have come to learn *so* much more in the past few years about the importance of vitamin D, which is also known as the "sunshine vitamin" in honor of the primary source of vitamin D for humans: the sun.

Once the vitamin D taken in through diet, supplementation, or sunlight, it is metabolized in the kidneys into its bioactive form (called 1,25-dihydroxyvitamin D, or 1,25(OH)2D for short) and it goes to work on a number of tissues, organs, and systems, of the body, as explained via research published in Nutrients [4]:

> ***"Vitamin D is a steroid hormone that is vitally important for all vertebrates****, including humans. Maintaining normal serum levels of calcium and phosphate is critically dependent on vitamin D. Vitamin D thus contributes to the well-being of the human body by* ***promoting a strong skeletal system, facilitating muscle movement, supporting the immune system, and optimizing cellular functions throughout the body.****"*

The vast benefits of vitamin D (which, again, we are just beginning to fully unravel) include:

- Stronger bones via increased calcium absorption (more on the relationship between vitamin D, vitamin K, and calcium coming up)

- Improved mood, reduced anxiety and depression
- Reduced risk of numerous chronic diseases associated with inflammation, including multiple sclerosis (MS), heart disease, type 1 diabetes, inflammatory bowel disease (IBD), rheumatoid arthritis, and more
- Reduced severity of, and faster recovery from, acute infections like COVID-19
- Faster, more sustainable weight loss

In addition to those impressive benefits, vitamin D promotes the healthy expression of nearly a *thousand* genes, representing about 3% of the entire genome, acting as what biologists call an "epigenetic" agent.

We could devote a whole chapter to epigenetics, which is the study of how physical changes (in this case, vitamin D supplementation) can affect the expression (or activity) of DNA.

"Epi" is a Greek-derived prefix that means "outside of" or "on top of," so "epigenetics" in clinical practice focuses on how to beneficially alter the activity of genes that already exist in the DNA by turning on health-promoting genes and turning off disease-causing genes.

From an anti-aging perspective, we want all the beneficial epigenetic action we can get. And vitamin D is a powerful epigenetic tool.

More from Nutrients:

> *"Vitamin D, or more specifically,* ***its biologically active form 1,25(OH)2D*** *[1,25-dihydroxyvitamin D], behaves like a steroid hormone,* ***influencing around 900 different genes or roughly 3% of the human genome****, either directly or indirectly…*
>
> *1,25(OH)2D is known to play a crucial role in calcium homeostasis, as well as in controlling blood pressure and electrolytes. Through VDRs,* ***1,25(OH)2D controls genes associated with energy metabolism, detoxification, immune function, and the maintenance of calcium homeostasis.****"*

As just one example of vitamin D's extraordinary benefits for immune function, take a gander at the now well-documented relationship between vitamin D status and COVID-19 severity, documented in a 10-study systematic review published via medical journal QJM [5]:

> *"For this study, systematic reviews and meta-analysis published from December 2019 to January 2022 presenting the impact of vitamin D supplementation on COVID-19 severity were screened and selected from PubMed and Google scholar...*
>
> ***The findings of this study show that vitamin D supplementation is effective in reducing the COVID-19 severity. Hence, vitamin D should be recommended as an adjuvant therapy for COVID-19.**"*

The second reason that we must pay so much attention to this steroid hormone is that vitamin D deficiency is *rampant* in the developed world. The reasons for widespread lack of vitamin D are many, including that we simply don't spend sufficient time outside soaking up healthy sunshine and, when we do, we often lather on the sunscreen that prevents the absorption of its rays.

Returning to Nutrients:

> ***"Vitamin D deficiency is a serious public health problem, affecting nearly 50% of the global population*****. Low serum levels of vitamin D are being associated with increased susceptibility to numerous health conditions, including respiratory infections, mental health, autoimmune diseases, and different cancer types."*

*I find that, in fact, not 50% but a shocking 90% of my LowTE Florida patients are deficient in vitamin D—in the Sunshine State, no less! So, it's my opinion that the percentage of the American population with vitamin D deficiency far exceeds the often-cited figure of 50%.

Vitamin D deficiency is particularly pronounced in the winter, when the sun is weaker and we spend less time outdoors, and it's more common in office workers and others who spend most of their time indoors.

According to most public health bodies, vitamin D levels between 30–100 ng/mL (75-250 nmol/L) are considered "normal," with anything below 30 being considered an insufficiency or deficiency.

However, it is my opinion, and increasingly the consensus of anti-aging medical practitioners on the front lines of clinical practice, that a vitamin D level around 30 ng/mL is far from optimal. My aim at LowTE Florida is to get my patients' vitamin D levels between 60-80 and then maintain that level. However, vitamin D is a fat-soluble vitamin, meaning that it may accumulate, and excess may not be excreted. So regular testing is critical. Like thyroid—you don't want too much, and you don't want too little!

Additionally, unlike other products that contain only vitamin D, our LowTE Florida vitamin D supplement contains complementary and critical vitamin K.

Here's why any vitamin D supplement worth its salt includes vitamin K and, in fact, why supplementing with D without including any K can be dangerous. Let's explore briefly an excerpt from an article titled "The Synergistic Interplay between Vitamins D and K for Bone and Cardiovascular Health: A Narrative Review," published in the International Journal of Endocrinology [6]:

> *"**Vitamins D and K** are **both** fat-soluble vitamins **and play a central role in calcium metabolism.** Vitamin D promotes the production of vitamin K-dependent proteins, which **require vitamin K for carboxylation in order to function properly...***
>
> *A growing body of **evidence suggests a synergistic effect of vitamin K combined with vitamin D...***
>
> *Animal and human studies suggest that optimal concentrations of both vitamin D and vitamin K are beneficial for bone and cardiovascular health."*

In layman's terms, the indispensable benefit of including vitamin K alongside vitamin D is that vitamin D enhances calcium absorption downstream. Increased calcium absorption, in turn, can be a health benefit or health risk depending on *where* it's stored.

To that end, vitamin K helps move calcium out of the blood vessels where it *doesn't* belong—where it can calcify and lead to atherosclerosis over time (the clinical term for scarring and hardening of the arteries which you definitely don't want)—and shuttle the K, instead, into the bones where it *does* belong to keep them strong and prevent osteoporosis.

Specifically, the form of vitamin K included in my LowTE Florida ADK supplement (menaquinone-7, or MK-7) is proven to be the most bioavailable form available for maximum absorption.

In particular, the benefits of vitamin K supplementation for heart health have been best demonstrated in the blood vessels of postmenopausal women, for example via the Journal of Thrombosis and Haemostasias [7]:

> ***"We investigated long-term effects of MK-7*** *(180 µg MenaQ7/day) supplementation* ***on arterial stiffness in a double-blind, placebo-controlled trial…***
>
> *After… MK-7 supplementation cfPWV (Carotid-femoral pulse wave velocity) and the Stiffness Index β significantly decreased in the total group, whereas distension, compliance, distensibility, Young's Modulus, and the local carotid PWV (cPWV) improved in women having a baseline Stiffness Index β above the median of 10.8. MK-7 decreased dp-ucMGP by 50% compared to placebo…* ***Long-term use of MK-7 supplements improves arterial stiffness in healthy postmenopausal women,*** *especially in women having a high arterial stiffness."*

It's for the sake of my patients' hearts and arteries that I include vitamin K in its most bioavailable form in my LowTE Florida ADK supplement. Wherever you source your sunshine vitamin, I advise all my patients to never take large vitamin D doses without accompanying vitamin K.

All the clinical data I've shared so far that went into crafting LowTE Florida ADK is realized in the real-life patients this supplement delivers to my patients, like Chris M.:

> *"**LowTE Florida ADK supplement has been a fantastic addition to my daily routine.** The combination of Vitamin A, Vitamin D3, and Vitamin K2 in this supplement has provided me with numerous health benefits. **I've noticed improvements in my bone health, immune function, and overall well-being.** The quality of the product is exceptional. I highly recommend LowTE Florida ADK supplement to anyone looking to improve their vitamin D deficiency."*

Diagnosing and correcting low vitamin D status is simple and extremely affordable, even on the most modest of budgets. I know because I help my patients do it every day. There's simply no excuse for a deficiency in this vitamin in the modern era—another failure of mainstream medicine that we ought to remedy as a society.

If you might be of the hundreds of millions of Americans with sub-optimal vitamin D levels (remember vitamin D deficiency, by many estimates, affects over 50% of the population) then, for the sake of your health, don't wait to correct your levels and enjoy the massive benefits of elevated levels of the sunshine vitamin. LowTE Florida ADK comes in 5,000 iu's and 10,000 iu's.

LowTE Florida Probiotic

You might not know that, at any given moment, your gut microbiome plays host to anywhere between 30 and 400 ***trillion*** (with a t!) living microorganisms—including as many as a thousand species of bacteria. In fact, there are actually 100 times more bacteria cells in your gut than human cells in your whole body.

Digest those staggering numbers for a moment!

All those microorganisms who have made themselves at home in your gut might sound scary at first, but there is, actually, a vital role for the *good* bacteria in our gut, which we don't just live alongside but absolutely need for many functions, including:

- Supplying cellular energy for the gut to do its metabolic work
- Breaking down food
- Synthesizing vitamins
- Eliminating other pathogenic bacteria, viruses, and fungi
- Detoxification

The key to optimal health, therefore, is boosting the numbers of beneficial bacteria while limiting the numbers of harmful bacteria, fungi, and viruses.

There's an eternal microscopic war in your gut, if you will, between the forces of health and illness, and our aim is to give the good guys the tools they need to thrive and win.

(This is a side note, but an important one; the centrality of beneficial gut bacteria to overall health is why you want to avoid the overuse of antibiotics, as they indiscriminately kill both harmful *and* helpful bacteria. In some cases, of course, of acute infection, antibiotics are necessary as a short-term treatment, but their use should be judicious and limited. It's my view, backed up by evidence, that the medical profession relies entirely too much on antibiotics as a frontline treatment, potentially doing more harm than good.)

It's difficult to exaggerate the importance of optimal gut health, as the scientific consensus is rapidly bearing down in recent years on the recognition that many, if not *most*, chronic health conditions (particularly chronic inflammatory, neurodegenerative, and autoimmune conditions) have their genesis in the gut.

For further elaboration, let's turn to the European Journal of Clinical Nutrition [8]:

> *"**Alteration in the levels of gut microbial metabolites,** such as SCFAs, ammonia, tryptophan, and histamine **have shown to be***

> ***associated,*** *directly or by breaking down into neuroactive catabolites* ***with various neurological conditions like Parkinson's disease (PD), anorexia nervosa (AN), Alzheimer's disease (AD), autism spectrum disorder (ASD), and chronic stress and depression…***
>
> *Given the tight interplay between enteric microbial symbionts and host immunity, efforts have focused on implementing various strategies targeting the gut microbiota to manage or prevent chronic diseases.* ***Clinical approaches to modify gut microbiota generally focus on*** *depleting overabundant members or the overall microbial load using antibiotics or antifungal agents, modulation through diet, or* ***supplementation with live microbes*** *(single or mixed species) …*
>
> *Over the past decade,* ***considerable evidence from both animal and human studies has accumulated showing a clear link between the gut microbiome in chronic diseases,*** *including inflammatory autoimmune disorders, gut inflammation-related disorders, and cardiometabolic diseases. It is increasingly clear that bacterial metabolites are at least in part, the key agents involved in the role of the gut microbiome on human health and among such metabolites, SCFAs appear to be the most important ones. Butyrate-producing bacteria are associated with lower risk of inflammatory autoimmune and cardiometabolic diseases, and also irritable bowel syndrome.* ***A number of therapeutic strategies to target the gut microbiome are possible."***

Unfortunately, the on-the-ground practice of frontline clinical care has not sufficiently caught up to this increasingly apparent and well-documented reality, as gut health remains woefully neglected in mainstream medicine.

To really get a healthcare provider to give the gut the attention it deserves, you need to see a specialist with a deeper understanding of it, like me.

Hopefully, in the future, as more and more evidence of the centrality of the gut to overall health emerges, and doctors receive more education in this long-neglected domain, the lack of mind paid to the microbiome will change, and gut health examinations will become components of standard wellness check-ups.

But, unfortunately, that's where the practice of mainline medicine is now.

At any rate, the reason my patients are so loyal is that we do things differently in my LowTE Florida practice, in that we base all our treatment protocols on the most cutting-edge research available. As the body of biomedical knowledge at our fingertips evolves, so does much of our approach to healthcare.

Using that mantra as our north star, we deliver superior results in the process, which is all that matters in the end.

Accordingly, I do *not* ignore gut health in my LowTE Florida practice. On the contrary, I make replenishing and healing the microbiome with vitality-enhancing bacteria a fundamental cornerstone of my approach to anti-aging healthcare.

The name of the gut health game from a therapeutic perspective, once again, is moving *in* beneficial bacteria and moving *out* the harmful bacteria and fungi to create a healthier, more functional, uninflamed microbiome.

That's what LowTE Florida Probiotic achieves. Each dose delivers a proprietary 60 mg blend of the following beneficial bacteria, commonly used to treat irritable bowel syndrome (IBS) inflammatory bowel disease (IBD), and numerous other conditions affecting the gut:

- Bifidobacterium longum
- Lactobacillus rhamnoses
- Lactobacillus acidophilus

LowTE Florida Probiotic is in a class above your standard, store-bought probiotic supplement, and here's why: unlike many probiotic supplements that the capsule opens in the stomach, which results in all the good microbiota being killed by the stomach acid and neutralizing any benefit, the patented capsule technology developed for LowTE Florida Probiotic causes the probiotics to be released in the beginning of the small intestines, where they are unleashed to do their critical work.

Once the therapeutic bacteria in LowTE Florida Probiotic are released into the intestines, they proliferate and flourish, replacing harmful bacteria and fungi like candida, and creating a microbiome that ultimately contributes to your overall health instead of detracting from it.

Substantial research backs up the therapeutic applications of each of the potent probiotic strains in LowTE Florida Probiotic—Bifidobacterium longum, Lactobacillus rhamnoses, and Lactobacillus acidophilus—for instance, via the American Journal of the Medical Sciences [9]:

> *"Probiotics are defined as living microorganisms, principally bacteria, which are safe for human consumption…* ***When ingested in sufficient quantities, probiotics have beneficial effects for human health, beyond basic nutrition****. These effects may result from suppression of pathogens and stimulation of probiotic growth that contributes to the nutrition and health of the gut.*
>
> *The major strains,* ***Lactobacillus (lacto.) acidophilus****, Lactobacillus casei* ***and various Bifidobacterium species, are the most dominant bacteria in the small and large intestine of humans*** *that can inhibit the growth of pathogenic microorganisms, through production of organic acids and bacteriocin. Theresa,* ***several strains of lactic acid bacteria (LAB) were reported to display stimulatory properties on cells of the innate immune system*** *in-vitro."*

One of the biggest medical discoveries of the past century, which is still unfolding, is the intimate and previously totally unknown connection between the gut and the brain.

It was formerly assumed (incorrectly) in the medical canon that the nervous system and the digestive system were wholly separate and independent, but we now know they are so closely connected that many now refer to the gut as the body's "second brain" because of the influence it exerts on the nervous system and vice versa. This phenomenon is often called the "brain-gut axis."

It stands to reason, then, that optimizing gut health through probiotic supplementation and diet would have a positive impact on mental health. And that's exactly what recent research has determined.

Let's survey an extensive literature review of over three dozen studies on the benefits of probiotic supplementation for brain health published via the Journal of Neurogastroenterology and Motility [10]:

> *"38 studies were included: 25 in animals and 15 in humans (2 studies were conducted in both). Most studies used Bifidobacterium (eg, B. longum, B. breve, and B. infantis) and Lactobacillus (e.g., L. helveticus, and L. rhamnoses), with doses between 10^8 and 10^{10} colony-forming units for 2 weeks in animals and 4 weeks in humans. These* ***probiotics showed efficacy in improving psychiatric disorder-related behaviors including anxiety, depression, autism spectrum disorder (ASD), obsessive-compulsive disorder, and memory abilities, including spatial and non-spatial memory.****"*

Supplementation with a high-quality product like LowTE Florida Probiotic, with its patented technology to deliver the good stuff directly into the intestinal tract, has been demonstrated to confer the following benefits:

- Remission of chronic gut conditions like IBS, IBD, Crohn's disease, ulcerative colitis, and chronic diarrhea
- Improvements in mental health conditions like depression and anxiety
- Improved cognition and memory
- Reductions in chronic inflammation

- Lowered LDL cholesterol levels (the "bad" cholesterol)
- A more functional, strengthened immune system
- Weight loss via improved fat metabolism

So, if you want to look and feel your best (mentally, emotionally, and physically) we've got to focus on getting your gut health in order. My commitment is that when you visit my LowTE Florida office, we'll get to work doing just that.

LowTE Florida patient Larissa B. shares her experience using our unique probiotic:

> *"I've ordered this item from this company many times. Always good."*
>
> *"As good or better than any other probiotic we've ever used—outstanding (noticeable differences directly attributable to this product, not just coincidental),"* chimes in LowTE patient Chris S.

LowTE Florida Methyl Factors+

Methylation is an enzyme-facilitated, critical biochemical process carried out constantly, day and night, while active or at rest, inside the body at the cellular level; you don't know that's it's going on because it occurs automatically and you can't consciously feel it, but around the clock methylation helps your body with:

- Regulation of gene expression (an activity called epigenetic modulation, an important but under-appreciated facet of anti-aging care that we'll dive into in detail coming up)
- Detoxification from heavy metals (lead, mercury, etc.)
- Protein regulation
- Cell metabolism
- Production of neurotransmitters critical for optimal mental health

...and more.

Put simply, if healthy methylation function breaks down, so does your health in myriad, potentially devastating ways.

And there is **one thing** that **can and does often go very wrong with methylation**: mutations of the gene that controls methylation by creating the enzyme that facilitates the process, which is called methylenetetrahydrofolate reductase (MTHFR).

In a huge (and I do mean *huge*) minority of the American population, verging on a majority, an MTHFR mutation is present in at least one of the two alleles (parts) of the gene, which can impair MTHFR enzyme activity and in turn impact multiple facets of physical and mental health, as explained by way of Psychology Today [11]:

> ***"Up to 40% of the population may have an MTHFR mutation of some kind****. The current data suggest that between 6 and 14% of Caucasians and about 2% of those of African descent probably have a more severe (two mutated alleles) version of the mutation. In Hispanics, this number may be as high as 21%...*
>
> ***Even having one mutated allele is associated with an increased risk of certain health problems****...*
>
> *The* ***mental health issues linked to having an MTHFR mutation [are] depression, bipolar disorder, schizophrenia, attention-deficit hyperactivity disorder (ADHD), or autism****.* ***MTHFR mutations also increase the risk of*** *several physical health problems, including but not limited to* ***cardiovascular disease and stroke, recurrent early miscarriage, migraine with aura, osteoporosis, and some cancers****."*

40% of the American population is afflicted with a methylation deficiency! Based on my clinical experience, I can confirm that this figure is in the ballpark.

Mutations of the MTHFR gene can affect your body's ability to synthesize bioavailable folate, riboflavin, B6, B12, and other B vitamins. In addition, MTHFR mutations can affect how your body processes and uses supplements or drugs, potentially nullifying their benefits.

When methylation isn't humming along as it's supposed to, the body fails to synthesize enough of these critical compounds, neurotransmitters, and proteins—many of which you are likely familiar with because of their demonstrable importance to maintaining good health:

- Cysteine
- Nitric oxide (NO)
- Serotonin
- Melatonin
- Coenzyme Q10
- Glutathione, aka the "master antioxidant"

If all those effects of methylation dysfunction sound dreadful, fret not; there's good news on two fronts:

- Testing for MTHFR mutations is easy and affordable via a simple blood test, which I make available my LowTE Florida office
- Supplementation with Methyl Factor+—along with a whole foods-based diet, regular exercise, and limited alcohol and caffeine intake—can reverse critical nutrient deficits in individuals with MTHFR mutations who require augmentation

Methyl Factors+ contains the following roster of nutrients that are often severely depleted in my patients with impaired methylation:

- Riboflavin (vitamin B2)
- Pyridoxine (vitamin B6)
- L-5-methyl-tetrahydrofolate (also called methyl folate or 5-MTHF). This is the potent methylated form of folate which is already bioavailable and ready to nourish your cells and tissues, bypassing the need for methylation that is impaired in those with MTHFR mutations.
- Methyl cobalamin (methylated B12). Like 5-MTHF, this is the pre-methylated form of critical vitamin B12, rendering it bioactive as soon as it passes through the digestive system.

- Trimethyl glycine (TMG). TMG is an amino acid derivative that facilitates greater methylation and stabilizes homocysteine levels in those with MTHFR mutations.

It's the bioavailable nature of each of these B-vitamin compounds, combined with the synergistic aspect of TMG, that gives LowTE Methyl Factors+ its competitive edge.

Verified owner Chris S. compares his experiences with Methyl Factors+ to other popular B-vitamin complexes: "Superior in ingredients to a similar product used with HRT pellets which we used for a couple of years previously. We now prefer LowTE Florida's similar formulations."

Simple and cost-effective, yet powerful and transformative, tweaks to your supplement regimen, diet, and movement habits can make profound improvements to your body's methylation status.

I make it a standard part of my initial examination with any patient to explore potential methylation problems and fix those through supplementation with Methyl Factors+ and lifestyle adjustments as necessary.

LowTE Florida Iodine+

Iodine is, paradoxically, at the same time one of the most neglected yet one of the most fundamental elements necessary for optimal human health.

It is, in my opinion, one of the great failures of modern medicine to not prioritize iodine optimization as an integral part of general healthcare.

Chances are high that you may have never even consciously considered the importance of dietary iodine. But it deserves far more attention than a passing mention, especially considering the dramatic and shocking iodine deficiency statistics that we'll explore coming up.

The all-important element iodine supports and enhances health in a variety of ways—perhaps most importantly for thyroid function, as explained by the National Institutes of Health [12]:

*"**Iodine is an essential component of the thyroid hormones** thyroxine (T4) and triiodothyronine (T3). **Thyroid hormones regulate many important biochemical reactions, including protein synthesis and enzymatic activity, and are critical determinants of metabolic activity.** They are also required for proper skeletal and central nervous system development in fetuses and infants"*

Because of iodine's well-documented thyroid-boosting properties, for many of my patients with iodine deficiency, LowTE Florida Iodine+ pairs spectacularly with bioidentical thyroid hormone extract for boosting the thyroid and reaping all of the consequent benefits.

I prescribe iodine to combat a variety of chronic and common health conditions, with overwhelming success in reducing symptom frequency and intensity. These include but are not limited to:

- Atherosclerosis (hardening of the arteries)
- High blood pressure
- Liver dysfunction
- Chronic fatigue
- Prostate problems
- Unwanted weight gain

Studies show optimized Iodine may support or reduce the following:

- Breast disease
- Fibrocystic breasts
- ADHD/ADD
- Excess Mucus
- Goiter/Thyroid disorders
- Ovarian disease
- Prostate disease
- Sebaceous cysts
- Vaginal infections
- Hemorrhoids
- Migraine head aches
- High blood pressure
- Infections

- Keloids

Iodine deficiency is a growing concern worldwide as it is in the United States. Since iodine was largely taken out of table salt and other food products years ago, this particularly pernicious nutritional deficit has returned to the developed world.

The United Nations and other public health bodies estimate that as many as **2 billion people worldwide suffer from untreated iodine deficiency**. That's roughly a quarter of the entire Earth population that needlessly experiences this deficiency, given that high-quality iodine supplementation is at our fingertips.

Achieving optimal iodine levels is problematic for populations that live far from the ocean and therefore eat limited amounts of seafood, the most abundant dietary source of minerals.

Soil depletion (the removal of vital minerals from the ground and therefore the crops they are grown in due to poor farming practices and other factors) also drives the iodine crisis: "The earth's soils contain varying amounts of iodine, which in turn affects the iodine content of crops. In some regions of the world, iodine-deficient soils are common, increasing the risk of iodine deficiency among people who consume foods primarily from those areas," notes the NIH.

Iodine deficiency is, again, most pronounced in regions far from the coasts as well as in cultures with diets lacking in animal products, as the foods with the most plentiful supplies of dietary iodine, in addition to ocean-sourced fish, include dairy and eggs.

Some foods (and a vanishing share of table salt products) in the developed world still contain supplemental iodine, which has helped alleviate some of the burden of iodine deficiency, but research suggests that much of the iodine in the foods and condiments we consume is not highly bioavailable, meaning it has limited therapeutic benefit.

It's my clinical experience, based on decades of nutritional consultations and blood testing, that dietary iodine intake alone is usually not enough to get levels into the ranges we want to see.

For this reason, LowTE Iodine+ is a staple in my patients' supplemental regimens. (LowTE Iodine+, in a single dose, supplies over 8,000% of the daily recommended minimum intake in a highly bioavailable package.)

My patients consistently report loving how they feel on LowTE Iodine+; surprising to me the most mentioned comment was on their increase in energy! I'll take it!

A note of caution: it's very easy—far too easy, as a matter of fact—to overdo it on iodine, especially if you have a pre-existing deficiency, which can have uncomfortable effects and sometimes negative health consequences.

It's essential, therefore, to consult with an experienced healthcare professional like me before beginning on an iodine protocol to avoid any issues.

LowTE Florida FreeTE

We've covered at great length in previous chapters the irreplaceable testosterone-boosting benefits of bioidentical hormone replacement therapy—which, as you've noted by now, is the bread and butter of the services I provide to my LowTE Florida patients.

In addition to bioidentical hormone replacement therapy, we also have available in our arsenal potent supplemental compounds that we can use to optimize T levels in men and women alike (and, equally importantly, balance the ratio of testosterone to estrogen) who need a leg-up in the androgen department.

To that end, we've developed a supplement containing the most powerful testosterone-boosting herbal extract known to man, used for millennia by folk medicine practitioners in India and beyond: tongkat ali (also known as E. Longifolia), the active component of our patented FreeTE product.

In some cases, we may use LowTE Florida FreeTE in combination with bioidentical testosterone therapy, while in other cases of more minor deficiencies we may be able to achieve optimal T levels with FreeTE alone. Each patient deserves an individualized treatment plan, and that's what I deliver at LowTE Florida.

The Patented FreeTE Active Ingredient: LJ100® Eurycoma Longifolia (Tongkat Ali)

We've covered the weight loss and stress-reduction benefits of tongkat ali previously, as it's one of the two major active components of another unique product I offer my patients: LowTE Florida Citru-Slim.

As we alluded to earlier, tongkat ali is also a potent testosterone booster with, again, thousands of years of use in folk medicine and a growing compendium of modern research to back it up.

Let's look, for example, at the following meta-analysis of numerous clinical trials testing tongkat ali's additive effects to testosterone counts, via Medicina [3], which found clinically significant improvements in T levels in both men with diagnosed low T (hypogonadism) and healthy testosterone levels:

> *"This study aims to* ***investigate the efficacy of E. longifolia*** *as a sole intervention* ***to increase testosterone levels in males...***
>
> *We conducted a systematic review and meta-analysis of randomized clinical trials (RCTs)...*
>
> *A total of nine studies was included in the systematic review. Five RCTs were included in the meta-analysis.* ***A significant improvement in total testosterone levels after E. longifolia treatment*** *was mostly reported* ***in both healthy volunteers and hypogonadal men.*** *The random model effect revealed a significant increase (SMD = 1.352, 95% CI 0.565 to 2.138, p = 0.001) in the total testosterone levels in men receiving E. longifolia*

supplementation, which was confirmed in the hypogonadism subgroup."

The specific form of the herbal extract that we use in LowTE Florida FreeTE, LJ100®, is a patented, highly bioavailable tongkat ali supplement produced by leading firm HP Ingredients, using exclusively herbs sourced from the Malaysian rainforest and backed by third-party lab testing for purity.

In my clinical opinion and based on my research, LJ100® is the cream of the crop when it comes to concentrated tongkat ali extracts, the real deal.

The proof is in the pudding: my patients love what FreeTE does for their libido, energy levels, and physical performance via increased testosterone levels and decreased stress hormone levels, and I'm confident you'll enjoy similar results if we determine that tongkat ali supplementation is right for you.

LowTE Florida Citru-Slim

Citru-Slim is one of our most highly reviewed and efficacious go-to weight loss supplements—an excellent adjunct to hormone replacement therapy in patients battling overweight/obesity and/or metabolic dysfunction—designed to confer the following benefits:

- Increased metabolism (calorie burning)
- Blood sugar regulation to prevent dangerous spikes
- Appetite suppression
- Reduced levels of the "stress hormone" cortisol
- Activation of the powerful anti-aging AMPK pathway (more on that later)
- Reduced levels of triglycerides (a harmful form of cholesterol)

My patients love Citru-Slim for three basic reasons: it's affordable, simple to take, and it delivers results.

Citru-Slim capsules are to be taken three times daily by mouth with meals and contain two active ingredients that we'll explore now.

Citru-Slim Active Ingredient #1: Bergamonte Full-Spectrum Citrus Bergamia Risso Fruit Extract

Bergamonte is the patented LowTE formulation of bergamot extract, an exotic citrus fruit with potent medicinal properties that originated in Southeast Asia but is now primarily grown in Italy.

By "full spectrum," we mean that Bergamonte contains *all* of the many medicinal compounds naturally occurring in the bergamot fruit, packed together in a highly concentrated form for maximum efficacy and bioavailability.

Instead of eating a massive amount of fruit, you reap all the benefits from a single, easy-to-swallow, convenient capsule.

Aside from simply tasting delicious (you might be familiar with bergamot as a popular and flavorful addition to tea), powerful bergamot fruit extract has numerous and wide-ranging health benefits, summarized below by way of an extensive literature review published in Food Science & Nutrition [13]:

> *"We summarize the effects of bergamot (extract, juice, essential oil, and polyphenolic fraction) on cardiovascular, bone, inflammatory, skin diseases, mood alteration, anxiety, pain, and stress. This review included a total of 31 studies (20 studies on humans with 1709 subjects and 11 in animals (rats and mice). In humans,* ***bergamot-derived extract (BE) exerts positive effects on hyperlipidemia*** *with an oral dose from 150 mg to 1000 mg/day of flavonoids administered from 30 to 180 days,* ***demonstrating an effect on body weight and in modulating total cholesterol, triglycerides, LDL, and HDL****. Studies in animals confirm* ***promising data on glucose control*** *(500/1000 mg/day of BE with a treatment lasting 30 days) are available in rats.* ***In animal models, bergamot*** *essential oil (BEO, 10 mg/kg or 20 mg/kg daily for 20*

weeks) ***increases bone volume, decreases psoriatic plaques, increases skin collagen content, and promotes hair growth.*** *"*

With all these versatile health benefits, bergamot is truly a miracle plant—a jewel in the vast inventory of plant-based medicine—which is why I directed our team to develop and patent our own highly concentrated and bioavailable bergamot extract, Bergamonte, for our LowTE Florida patients to benefit from.

Citru-Slim Active Ingredient #2: Adapticort Eurycoma Longifolia Extract

The second active ingredient in Citru-Slim is Adapticort, a patented, high-potency extract of *Eurycoma Longifolia*, an herb with thousands of years of use in traditional medicine, also known in popular parlance by a variety of other names, such as "tongkat ali," "longjack," or "Malaysian ginseng."

We standardize all Adapticort supplements to contain 22% active eurypeptides and 40% Glyco Saponins—the "good stuff" in tongkat ali that lends its therapeutic anti-aging properties, which we'll explore in detail now.

The first and most well-known benefit of tongkat ali is increased testosterone paired with decreased cortisol (stress hormone) levels, explained through research published in the medical journal Molecules [14]:

> *"Eurycomanone, the major quassinoid in the* ***E. longifolia root extract, significantly increased testosterone production on a dose-dependent manner*** *at 0.1, 1.0 and 10.0 μM (p < 0.05).* ***It enhanced testosterone steroidogenesis*** *at the rat testicular Leydig's cells* ***by inhibiting aromatase conversion of testosterone to estrogen,*** *and may also involve in phosphodiesterase inhibition at a high concentration."*

Aromatase is an enzyme that, as noted above, converts testosterone into estrogen—often to devastating effects in both men and women in cases of diagnosable testosterone deficiency.

The greater the aromatase enzyme activity, the lower testosterone levels fall, which represents one of the biggest culprits of low T in older men and menopausal women. The above study shows that **the bioactive compounds in tongkat ali inhibit, or suppress, the conversion or testosterone to estrogen, thereby increasing free testosterone levels**.

In addition to the treasure-trove of health benefits that elevated testosterone delivers to patients who need it—which we've explored at length in previous chapters—higher testosterone by way of bioidentical hormone replacement therapy at LowTE Florida and **tongkat ali supplementation also reduces cortisol levels**.

High cortisol stress hormone levels, , indicate high levels of physical or emotional stress, and may also point to a chronic condition such as adrenal insufficiency or Cushing's syndrome.

Stress and the stress hormones are testosterone killers; the inverse relationship between cortisol and testosterone levels (meaning lower cortisol levels result in higher testosterone levels and vice versa) is well-documented, as evidenced by way of the Journal of the International Society of Sports Nutrition [15]:

> ***"A negative relationship exists between the hormones cortisol and testosterone****. Bambino and Hsueh (1981) showed a direct inhibitory effect of high doses of glucocorticoids upon testicular Leydig cell function in rats, which resulted in a decrease in the production of testosterone. Cumming et al. (1983) found a similar relationship in humans, using pharmacological doses of cortisol to induce a decrease in testosterone production."*

In applied practice, the key is to figure out what's causing these cortisol spikes and how to reduce them.

I see elevated cortisol levels and corresponding low testosterone levels all too often in my LowTE Florida clinical practice. Reversing the ratio to restore healthy T levels and reduce cortisol levels is a key facet of my anti-aging strategy.

(In the upcoming section on my patented LowTE Florida testosterone booster, FreeTE, we'll dive into tongkat ali's potent pro-testosterone properties in greater detail.)

In addition to lowering cortisol levels and increasing testosterone levels, research indicates that tongkat ali potentially:

- Boosts libido (sex drive)
- Increases fertility
- Treats erectile dysfunction
- Increases lean muscle mass

Citru-Slim Research

As with all the LowTE products that I recommend to my patients, Citru-Slim has a cornucopia of research to back up its therapeutic utility.

In one study [16], researchers split participants into three groups, giving them either a placebo, 650 mg of Bergamonte BPE-Complex daily, or 1,300 mg of Bergamonte BPE-Complex daily for four months.

At the end of the four-month study period, here is what they found that Bergamonte BPE-Complex supplementation achieved compared to the placebo group:

- Decreased LDL and triglyceride (bad cholesterol) levels
- Increased HDL (good cholesterol) levels
- Reduced fasting blood sugar
- Reduced ghrelin (aka the "hunger hormone") levels
- Reduced body weight and body-mass index by up to 14.9% and 15.9%, respectively
- Increased adiponectin (a protein hormone that facilitates fatty acid breakdown and blood sugar control via activation of the AMPK signaling pathway*) levels by around 20%.

*As promised earlier, it's worth pausing here to elaborate a little bit on how the AMPK pathway works and why it's important for metabolic health and healthy weight loss, especially in older patients as AMPK activity tends to decline over time.

For a brief exploration of AMPK and its beneficial impacts on weight management, let's turn to Life Extension Magazine [17]:

"AMPK is found inside every cell and serves as a master energy sensor. Its activity level influences body fat composition and how long you'll live.

During their investigations, scientists discovered that boosting AMPK resulted in an unexpected benefit: the reduction of abdominal fat.

*Their findings made sense. Here's why. As we age, **cellular AMPK activity decreases and as a result, weight gain often follows**.*

*Excess weight, particularly in the abdominal region, accelerates aging processes. **Boosting AMPK activity results in a healthier metabolic status, which can lead to less fat production**.*

These findings were recently confirmed in a pair of human clinical trials. Researchers activated AMPK using two natural compounds. The result was a significant drop in abdominal fat.

*The first study showed that **abdominal fat deposits fell by 11%**. In the second study, **scientists observed a significant reduction in harmful inflammation**, which can contribute to weight gain."*

Similarly, significant research backs up Adapticort's proven capacity to reduce the "stress hormone" cortisol. In one study, 64 participants received either 200 mg/day of Adapticort or a placebo.

Here are the results, both in objective (data-driven) and subjective (how the trial participants reported feeling) terms:

- Cortisol levels fell by an average of 16% in the Adapticort group
- Testosterone levels rose by 37% in the Adapticort group

- Self-reported feelings of tension, anger, and confusion fell in Adapticort group by 11%, 12%, and 15%, respectively

Many of my LowTE patients to whom I recommend Citru-Slim in convenient capsule form for weight loss, appetite control, reduced stress, and increased testosterone notice the benefits in as little as a week of taking the product.

LowTE Florida Sleep Deep

We talked at length in a previous chapter about the devastating impacts on hormone health, and health in general, caused by insufficient sleep. I and most other healthcare experts define optimal slumber as 7-9 hours of uninterrupted sleep, with rare exceptions for so-called "super sleepers" who, based on genetics, can function well on less sleep.

Most of those who seek my counsel and care at LowTE Florida (and likely you as well) don't get 7-9 hours of restful sleep on a nightly basis. Some don't get anywhere close to that.

Therefore, helping my patients achieve optimal sleep habits is a pillar of my overall approach to anti-aging care.

With that goal in mind, my team has developed LowTE Florida Sleep Deep, our flagship sleep-enhancing supplement, crafted with no fewer than five proven ingredients that synergistically promote longer, more restful, uninterrupted sleep.

Sleep Deep Active Ingredient #1: Melatonin

The importance of melatonin to overall hormone health and the impressive benefits that it confers to numerous facets of anti-aging health, including most notably facilitating longer-lasting, more replenishing sleep, which is the reason it's included in LowTE Florida Deep Sleep.

Sleep Deep Active Ingredient #2: GABA (Gamma-Aminobutyric Acid)

Gamma-aminobutyric acid (GABA) is the brain's main inhibitor neurotransmitter, meaning that it slows and calms the nervous system for relaxation and sleep. In layman's terms, GABA directs the body's natural "rest and digest" functions, which includes the facilitation of healthy sleep.

In our over-stimulated, over-caffeinated, overworked world, relaxing GABA is more of a treasure than ever.

In a clinical trial published in the Journal of Clinical Neurology [18], researchers gave three dozen volunteers battling insomnia GABA supplementation and recorded its effects on sleep, finding it both efficacious and (unlike many prescription sleep aids) without any notable side effects:

> *"After 4 weeks of treatment* ***the sleep latency had decreased, and the sleep efficacy had increased only in the GABA treatment group...***
>
> ***The findings of this study suggest that... GABA can be used to reduce sleep latency and improve subjective sleep quality without serious adverse effects.*** *Because it is a naturally extracted substance without severe adverse events... GABA may be widely administered as a supplement to improve sleep health in the general population."*

Sleep Deep Active Ingredient #3: Lemon Balm Extract (Melissa officinalis)

Melissa officinalis, a member of the mint family known commonly as "lemon balm," is a vastly underrated sleep aid that delivers powerful results like prescription sleep aids—without, again, the same risk of dependence and potentially extreme negative side effects.

In a randomized placebo-controlled trial, in addition to finding that lemon balm extract relieved anxiety and depression, the scholars also lauded its therapeutic value for improving sleep quality, via Integrative Medicine Research [19]:

> *"**Melissa officinalis (lemon balm)** is known as a heart tonic and removes palpitations. It **has** also anxiolytic and antidepressant effects **and improves sleep quality**. It reduces palpitation in anxious patients... Using the standard form of Melissa officinalis (Cyracos), mild to moderate anxiety and sleep disturbances are reported to be improved."*

Sleep Deep Active Ingredient #4: Shoden® Ashwagandha

One of the principles I abide by in my clinical practice is that we, as all kinds of healthcare providers, ought to have the humility to draw from the wisdom of ancient cultures when the empirical evidence suggests it's appropriate. In many cases, traditional medicine was ahead of its time.

Such is the case with ashwagandha, an herb that has been used for thousands of years as a staple of Ayurvedic (ancient Indian) folk medicine. In recent years, Western medicine has confirmed its powerful therapeutic properties, including for sleep, via clinical research, such as that below by way of the Journal of Ethnopharmacology [20]:

> *"We performed a randomized, parallel-group, stratified design, placebo-controlled study. A total of 80 eligible participants, 40 in Arm-A (healthy) and 40 in Arm-B (insomnia) were assigned to two groups, either Ashwagandha or placebo and studied for 8-weeks...*
>
> ***In both healthy and insomnia subjects, there was a significant improvement in the sleep parameters in the Ashwagandha root extract supplemented group**. The improvement was found more significant in insomnia subjects than healthy subjects...*
>
> ***The present study confirms that Ashwagandha root extract can improve sleep quality and can help in managing insomnia.***

Ashwagandha root extract was well tolerated by all the participants irrespective of their health condition and age."

Based on the quantitative data collected in the study, patients receiving ashwagandha supplementation fell asleep faster, stayed asleep longer, and experienced more restorative sleep than the control group.

And improved sleep quality barely scratches the tip of the iceberg in terms of the potent therapeutic benefits of ashwagandha, which also include improved cognitive function, reduced inflammation, chronic pain relief, increased testosterone, and many others.

Shoden® Ashwagandha, which I use in LowTE Sleep Deep for maximum absorption and benefit is a highly bioactive formulation of the extract from NutriSciences Innovations.

Sleep Deep Active Ingredient #5: L-Theanine

L-theanine is a legendary amino acid best known for lending green tea its relaxing, sedating qualities that complement so nicely the caffeine boost.

(It's been proven that green tea increases alpha brain wave activity, associated with greater creativity and relaxation, and that's because of its l-theanine content. If you're a green tea drinker and have noticed the simultaneous, seemingly contradictory sensation of increased alertness and increased relaxation after green tea, you can thank the caffeine and l-theanine combination.)

The amino acid l-theanine has a proven track record in clinical research of reducing anxiety, improving immune system function, reducing blood pressure, and potentially reducing cancer risk.

In addition to this cornucopia of benefits, l-theanine is also shown to improve sleep. In one study published via Pharmaceutical Biology [21], l-theanine, in combination with another Sleep Deep ingredient we've already discussed, GABA, demonstrated remarkable sleep-enhancing benefits:

*"**GABA/l-theanine mixture** (100/20 mg/kg) **showed a decrease in sleep latency** (20.7 and 14.9%) and an **increase in sleep duration** (87.3 and 26.8%) compared to GABA or theanine alone. **GABA/l-theanine mixture led to a significant increase in rapid eye movement** (REM) (99.6%) and non-REM (NREM) (20.6%) **compared to controls.** The use of GABA/l-theanine mixture rather than GABA or l-theanine alone restored to normal levels sleep time and quality in the arousal animal model. The administration of GABA/l-theanine led to increased expression of GABA and the glutamate GluN1 receptor subunit."*

So, as the above research demonstrates, each of these individual Sleep Deep compounds (L-theanine, GABA, lemon balm extract, ashwagandha, and melatonin) facilitates improved, longer-lasting, more restful sleep. In synergistic combination, however, they produce even more profound benefits for my LowTE Florida patients than any one of them could on their own.

"Excellent," "very good," and "very efficient" are some of the descriptors offered by real-life LowTE Florida patients who have given Sleep Deep a chance, all available to peruse at our website, LowTEFlorida.com.

Money-Back Guarantee

One point of extreme (and well-deserved, if I might be so bold) pride that I take in each of my meticulously developed LowTE Florida supplements is the no-nonsense, no-strings-attached, ironclad money-back guarantee that I offer all my patients.

Here it is:

"Your purchases from LowTE Florida are always risk-free. If you're unhappy with your purchase for any reason at all, contact us within 60 days of your purchase and we will refund 100% of your money back. Take advantage of our guarantee if you're unsure whether a particular product is right for you: buy the product and then decide.

If it doesn't meet your highest expectations, email us at info@lowteflorida.com or call 888-791-4520.

Yes, it's really that simple! We will gladly refund 100% of your order, no questions asked, no attempt to dissuade you or sell you something else.

Yes, it's really that simple! If you have any questions about your order, please email us and we will be happy to assist you!"

To emphasize, we will never make you fill out any lengthy questionnaires or give you the run-around. If you aren't fully satisfied, we will refund your money, period. That's how confident I am, based on years of positive feedback from satisfied patients, that my LowTE Florida supplements deliver the results we promise.

My team is also committed to helping you out with any questions or concerns you might have regarding our products, including regarding dosing, health applications, what time of day is best to take any given supplement, etc.

> *"Customer service was always quick to take care of the problem and is very professional and polite. Thank you for your great service,"* raves LowTE Florida patient Deane S.

One last note: we regularly feature discounts and promotions for our wide range of LowTE Florida products, including the ones mentioned here and more, so don't be a stranger to https://lowteflorida.com/store/!

References

[1] Scientific American. (2011). Dirt Poor: Have Fruits and Vegetables Become Less Nutritious? Scientific American. https://www.scientificamerican.com/article/soil-depletion-and-nutrition-loss/

[2] Licznerska, B. and Baer-Dubowska, W. (2016). Indole-3-Carbinol and Its Role in Chronic Diseases. Advances in Experimental Medicine and Biology. https://pubmed.ncbi.nlm.nih.gov/27671815/

[3] Leisegang, K, Finelli, R., et al. (2022). Eurycoma longifolia (Jack) Improves Serum Total Testosterone in Men: A Systematic Review and Meta-Analysis of Clinical Trials. Medicina. https://www.ncbi.nlm.nih.gov/pmc/articles/PMC9415500/

[4] Mavar, M., Soric, T., et al. (2024). The Power of Vitamin D: Is the Future in Precision Nutrition through Personalized Supplementation Plans? Nutrients. https://www.mdpi.com/2072-6643/16/8/1176

[5] Shah, K., Varna, P. (2022). Does vitamin D supplementation reduce COVID-19 severity?: a systematic review. QJM. https://pubmed.ncbi.nlm.nih.gov/35166850/

[6] Van Ballegooijen, A., Pilz, S., et al. (2017). "The Synergistic Interplay between Vitamins D and K for Bone and Cardiovascular Health: A Narrative Review." International Journal of Endocrinology. https://www.ncbi.nlm.nih.gov/pmc/articles/PMC5613455/

[7] Knapen, M., Braam, L. (2015). Menaquinone-7 supplementation improves arterial stiffness in healthy postmenopausal women. A double-blind randomised clinical trial. Journal of Thrombosis and Haemostasis. https://pubmed.ncbi.nlm.nih.gov/25694037/

[8] Vijay, A., Valdes, A. (2022). Role of the gut microbiome in chronic diseases: a narrative review. European Journal of Clinical Nutrition. https://www.ncbi.nlm.nih.gov/pmc/articles/PMC8477631/

[9] Jebur, M. (2010). Therapeutic efficacy of Lactobacillus acidophilus against bacterial isolates from burn wounds. American Journal of the Medical Sciences. https://www.ncbi.nlm.nih.gov/pmc/articles/PMC3338227/

[10] Wang, H., Lee, I., et al. (2016). Effect of Probiotics on Central Nervous System Functions in Animals and Humans: A Systematic Review. Journal of Neurogastroenterology and Motility. https://pubmed.ncbi.nlm.nih.gov/27413138/

[11] Stein, T. (2014). "A Genetic Mutation That Can Affect Mental & Physical Health." Psychology Today. https://www.psychologytoday.com/us/blog/the-integrationist/201409/genetic-mutation-can-affect-mental-physical-health

[12] National Institutes of Health. (n.d.) Iodine. National Institutes of Health. https://ods.od.nih.gov/factsheets/Iodine-HealthProfessional/

[13] Perna, S., Spadaccini, D., et al. (2019). Efficacy of bergamot: From anti-inflammatory and anti-oxidative mechanisms to clinical applications as preventive agent for cardiovascular morbidity, skin diseases, and mood alterations. Food Science & Nutrition. https://pubmed.ncbi.nlm.nih.gov/30847114/

[14] Rehman, S., Choe, K., et al. (2016). Review on a Traditional Herbal Medicine, Eurycoma longifolia Jack (Tongkat Ali): Its Traditional Uses, Chemistry, Evidence-Based Pharmacology and Toxicology. Molecules. https://www.ncbi.nlm.nih.gov/pmc/articles/PMC6274257/

[15] Brownlee, K., Moore, A. (2005). Relationship Between Circulating Cortisol and Testosterone: Influence of Physical Exercise. Journal of the International Society of Sports Nutrition. https://www.ncbi.nlm.nih.gov/pmc/articles/PMC3880087/

[16] Citru-Slim Powerpoint. (20220). LowTE Florida. https://lowteflorida.com/wp-content/uploads/2022/03/CitruSlim-PowerPoint-October-2022.pdf

[17] Whitman, S. (2023). Boost AMPK To Reduce Abdominal Fat. Life Extension Magazine. https://www.lifeextension.com/magazine/2017/ss/boost-ampk-to-reduce-abdominal-fat

[18] Byun, J., Sin, Y., et al. (2018). Safety and Efficacy of Gamma-Aminobutyric Acid from Fermented Rice Germ in Patients with Insomnia Symptoms: A Randomized, Double-Blind Trial. Journal of Clinical Neurology. https://www.ncbi.nlm.nih.gov/pmc/articles/PMC6031986/

[19] Ranjbar, M., Firoozabadi, A., et al. (2018). Effects of Herbal combination (Melissa officinalis L. and Nepeta menthoides Boiss. & Buhse) on insomnia severity, anxiety and depression in insomniacs: Randomized placebo controlled trial. Integrative Medicine Research. https://www.ncbi.nlm.nih.gov/pmc/articles/PMC6303415/

[20] Langade, D., Thakare, V., et al. (2021). Clinical evaluation of the pharmacological impact of ashwagandha root extract on sleep in healthy volunteers and insomnia patients: A double-blind, randomized, parallel-group, placebo-controlled study. Journal of Ethnopharmacology. https://pubmed.ncbi.nlm.nih.gov/32818573/

[21] Kim, S., Jo, K., et al. (2019). GABA and l-theanine mixture decreases sleep latency and improves NREM sleep. Pharmaceutical Biology. https://www.ncbi.nlm.nih.gov/pmc/articles/PMC6366437/

[22] Sears, M. (2013). Chelation: Harnessing and Enhancing Heavy Metal Detoxification—A Review. The Scientific World Journal.

[23] Jepson, R., Mihaljevic, L, et al. (2004). Cranberries for preventing urinary tract infections. Cochrane Database of Systematic Reviews. https://pubmed.ncbi.nlm.nih.gov/15106157/

[24] Achufusi, T., Pellegrini, M. (2024). Milk Thistle. StatPearls. https://www.ncbi.nlm.nih.gov/books/NBK541075/

[] Giordano, D., Corrado, F., et al. (2011). Effects of myo-inositol supplementation in postmenopausal women with metabolic syndrome: a perspective, randomized, placebo-controlled study. Menopause. https://pubmed.ncbi.nlm.nih.gov/20811299/

[] Fischer, L., DaCosta, K. (2007). Sex and menopausal status influence human dietary requirements for the nutrient choline. American Journal of Clinical Nutrition. https://pubmed.ncbi.nlm.nih.gov/17490963/

Chapter XI
Beyond HRT: The Other Crucial Wellness Factors Never to Be Ignored

Anti-aging regimens like targeted supplementation and bioidentical hormone replacement therapy, as we've laid out in detail, are powerful and, in fact, indispensable tools to combat the aging process and keep your mind and body in tip-top shape.

The immense value of such interventions—BHRT, thyroid optimization and nutritional supplementation—is obviously why I prioritize their use in my LowTE Florida practice.

However, the reality is that there is no medical or supplemental substitute for any of the following anti-aging lifestyle practices:

- Healthy diet
- Optimal sleep (both quality and quantity)
- Minimizing and regulating stress
- Eliminating exposure to hormone-disrupting toxins

Any healthcare provider who neglects or downplays the vital importance of any of the above in their advice to you, the patient, is not deserving of your time or money; getting these habits in order is non-negotiable as we commence other therapeutic interventions like bioidentical hormone replacement.

So, let's give them their due by surveying each of these anti-aging regimens one-by-one, with practical steps you can take in each domain to give your health a massive upgrade.

Wellness Factor #1: The Vital Role of Nutrition in Anti-Aging Healthcare

What if I told you the single greatest health threat in the modern world is not something lurking out there in the dangerous external world, but right at home in your food pantry?

There's no sugar-coating it: the standard American diet (appropriately acronymized to SAD) is a total mess. No one is winning the great game of life on a diet heavy on processed foods full of added sugars and harmful vegetable oils and largely depleted of nutrients.

Chronic inflammation? Unwanted weight gain? Anxiety and depression? Poor diet is often the ultimate primary driver of these chronic conditions.

A nutrient-rich, macronutrient-balanced diet, on the other hand, is a veritable Fountain of Youth. A wise ancient, the Greek physician Hippocrates (from whose name we derive the Hippocratic Oath, our north star as healthcare clinicians: "First, do no harm") once said: "Let food be thy medicine."

Unfortunately, at some point in our modern world, we collectively abandoned that lesson, largely but not entirely because of the pharmaceutical and medical industries that would rather focus on expensive drugs than basic (and inexpensive) practices like eating well to improve health.

Doctors-in-training in American medical school, as evidence of this, receive an appallingly microscopic amount of nutrition training. Let this data from the Harvard T.H. Chan School of Public Health [1] on the state of nutrition education in medical schools sink in:

> *"Despite the connection between poor diet and many preventable diseases,* ***only about one-fifth of American medical schools require students to take a nutrition course****, according to David Eisenberg, adjunct associate professor of nutrition at Harvard T.H. Chan School of Public Health. He discussed the topic May 8,*

2017 on PBS NewsHour in a segment that featured the Healthy Kitchens, Healthy Lives program that he founded. Co-sponsored by Harvard Chan School and the Culinary Institute of America, the program provides doctors and other health professionals with a crash course in how to build food and nutrition into their medical practices to improve health.

Today, most medical schools in the United States teach less than 25 hours of nutrition over four years*. The fact that less than 20 percent of medical schools have a single required course in nutrition, it's a scandal. It's outrageous. It's obscene,' Eisenberg told NewsHour."*

Less than *one out of five medical schools* in the United States requires students to complete *even a single course in nutrition*, even though diet is indisputably the single most important facet of health, an ancient truth that we've recognized as a species for thousands of years. It boggles the mind and shocks the conscience.

The good news is that, from my unique perspective within the healthcare industry, I see a resurgence in our collective conscious awareness of the vital role that nutrition plays in our mental, physical, and spiritual health.

So, what are Americans eating that is so terrible? The so-called standard American diet (SAD) consists of ultra-processed industrial foods strip-mined of all their nutrition, added sugar, high-fructose corn syrup and other artificial sweeteners, and seed oils and other synthetic fats.

You might sometimes see SAD also called the "Western diet"—although that label is a bit of an anachronism, as these harmful eating patterns have now been exported across the world by multinational food corporations (KFC, McDonald's, etc.) and pop culture. Industrialized food systems, it's sad to say, have made the Western diet the world's diet. And we've all paid the price in terms of reduced quality of life, shortening lifespans (for the first time in modern history life expectancy in the U.S. recently fell), and ballooning healthcare costs. Consider the absurdity of America devoting a full 20% of our annual GDP, $4.1

trillion, our national treasure that could otherwise be spent on so many other priorities, with little to no attention given by our public health bodies to cleaning up our diets, the simplest and most obvious solution to correcting course.

The U.S. Institute of Medicine [2] below summarizes well and succinctly the essential characteristics of SAD and its effects at the population level on public health:

> *"In the United States,* ***poor diet*** *was once associated with undernutrition. Today it* ***is more often associated with excess, particularly excesses in calories, saturated fats, trans fats, added sugars, and sodium.*** *The poor diets and sedentary lifestyles of the American public have led to high rates of obesity, overweight, and diet-related chronic diseases, including cardiovascular disease (CVD), hypertension, dyslipidemia, type 2 diabetes, osteoporosis, and certain types of cancer (HHS/USDA, 2005a).* ***It has been estimated that poor diet quality and physical inactivity contributed to approximately 16.6 percent* of U.S. deaths in 2000, compared to 14 percent in 1990."***

*Although I have not undertaken the rigorous clinical research to prove this claim, it's my experience that the sub-par diet of the general American public contributes to *much* more than 16% of deaths as of 2024, as we now know, again, that diet is the single most important factor for health and longevity.

Furthermore, those numbers are from the turn of the millennium; the SAD problem has certainly not gotten better in the last quarter century.

A chronic, steady SAD, as explained by the Scandinavian Journal of Pain [3], wreaks havoc on body weight, muscle mass, and bone density. It also, perhaps most importantly, fuels chronic systemic inflammation, the under-appreciated deadliness of which we have discussed in a previous chapter:

*"**Chronic consumption of the SAD increased fat mass, decreased lean mass and reduced bone mineral density. SAD-fed rats had increased leptin levels and pro-inflammatory cytokines** in peripheral blood serum. Following CFA administration, mechanical sensitivity was assessed, and recovery was delayed significantly in SAD-fed animals...*

In males, the SAD had a greater effect on bone mineral density and body composition. Long-term consumption of the SAD resulted in elevated microglial staining in the dorsal horn of the spinal cord...

*These data suggest **that poor quality diet may increase susceptibility to chronic pain** due to persistent peripheral and central immune system activation. **Furthermore, consumption of a diet that is high in carbohydrates and omega-6 polyunsaturated fatty acid is likely to lead to protracted recovery following trauma or surgical procedures.**"*

The good news is that, with our current level of knowledge in the domains of nutrition and human physiology, as well as the large diversity of foods now available in the developed world, tailoring your diet to optimize your health has never been easier—if you have the right guidance and the proper self-discipline to attain it.

First, before we dive into what you should be eating, let's survey some of the food products that you want to avoid like the plague.

Everybody's personalized approach to optimal nutrition, from both a macronutrient and micronutrient standpoint, will vary somewhat depending on unique genetics and fitness goals. However, it's my professional opinion, based on the available research, that everyone should swear off these food products once and for all and never look back because they simply do not belong in the human diet, period:

- **High-fructose corn syrup (HFCS)**. There's not much in our processed food supply that's more prevalent than wholly unnatural high-fructose corn syrup (HFCS), an artificial food product first developed for human consumption in the 1970s and synthesized by extracting highly concentrated glucose and fructose molecules from corn starch.

Regular consumption of HFCS (which is found in everything from soda to fruit juices to snack bars to oatmeal) is linked to metabolic dysfunction, obesity, chronic inflammation, heart disease, and cancer.

"The increased consumption of fructose in the average diet through sweeteners such as high-fructose corn syrup (HFCS) and sucrose has resulted in negative outcomes in society through producing a considerable economic and medical burden on our healthcare system. Ingestion of fructose chronically has contributed to multiple health consequences, such as insulin resistance, obesity, liver disorders, and diabetes," reports the Diabetes, Metabolic Syndrome and Obesity [4].

In other words, virtually every major cause of death in the developed world is associated with HFCS.

- **Processed sugar**. Here's a challenge I issue to all of my patients with questions about processed sugar consumption: the next time you visit the grocery store, when you're considering a processed food item—whether it be cereal or yogurt or so-called energy bars—take a hard look at the nutrition label before you toss it in the cart.

  The FDA requires that not just total sugar content, but all *added* sugars must be clearly declared on the package.

  You'll be shocked by what you find.
- **Seed oil**. Although seed oils are exceptionally cheap to produce (the reason they are so heavily marketed to the public), they are entirely synthetic substances that never existed in the human diet until the last half-century or so.

  We are only now just beginning to understand the hell that seed oils unleash on human health, which include wreaking havoc on the microbiome, promoting chronic inflammation, disruption of the delicate omega 3 to omega 6 ratio (seed oils being almost entirely omega 6 fatty acids), etc.—in other words, most of the negative upstream health deficits leading to chronic illness that we've already discussed in this book.

Common seed oils to ditch include grapeseed, sunflower, and canola. Toss them out with extreme prejudice.

- **Margarine**. If you're old enough to remember, like I am, the time many decades ago when margarine was aggressively touted by public health officials and marketers as a "healthy" alternative to butter or other natural cooking oils, this one's for you. My, oh my, how times have changed! As with the health effects of so many other products (let's not forget the time in distant history when cigarettes came doctor-recommended), we missed the mark big time on margarine, which we now recognize as a major threat to heart and metabolic health.

  From the Cleveland Clinic[5]: "Margarine may contain trans-fat, which raises LDL (bad) cholesterol, lowers HDL (good) cholesterol and makes blood platelets stickier, increasing heart disease risk. Margarine containing hydrogenated or partially hydrogenated oils contain trans fats and should be avoided."
- **Pesticides**. In our modern world, it's virtually impossible to totally avoid pesticides, which are found in basically every food item imaginable to one degree or another. Even foods labeled "organic" and adorned with the iconic USDA Organic seal of approval often turn up positive results when they're tested for pesticides.

  Among many negative health effects, many commercially-used pesticides are potent endocrine disruptors, meaning they throw off the delicate balance of the hormone system, potentially negating any progress you might make from bioidentical hormone replacement therapy and other treatments to optimize and balance hormones—not good.

  But, because they're ubiquitous in the food supply, you'd go crazy (and hungry) if you really tried to avoid pesticides altogether. The name of the game, therefore, is to *limit* your exposure to pesticides rather than hope to eliminate them entirely.

To that end, Environmental Working Group (EWG) [6] offers some insights and basic rules for minimizing pesticide exposure:

*"This year, EWG determined that **75 percent of all conventional fresh produce sampled had residues of potentially harmful pesticides. But for items on the Dirty Dozen, a whopping 95 percent of samples contain pesticides**...*
Of the 46 items included in our analysis, these 12 fruits and vegetables were most contaminated with pesticides:

1. Strawberries
2. Spinach
3. Kale, collard and mustard greens
4. Grapes
5. Peaches
6. Pears
7. Nectarines
8. Apples
9. Bell and hot peppers
10. Cherries
11. Blueberries
12. Green beans."

This isn't to say that you can't eat these foods—spinach and blueberries are highly nutritious if we look beyond the pesticide contamination issue—but rather that, if you do eat these fruits and veggies, it's a good idea to clean them thoroughly. I'd recommend letting them soak in a container of baking soda for at least an hour or two, as this process has been demonstrated to remove a large portion of pesticide residue.

On the other side of the ledger, the EWG identified the "Clean Fifteen"—the 15 cleanest produce products with the least detectable amounts of pesticides:

"These 15 types of produce had the lowest amounts of pesticide residues, according to EWG's analysis of the most recent USDA data.

1. Avocados

2. Sweet corn
3. Pineapple
4. Onions
5. Papaya
6. Sweet peas (frozen)
7. Asparagus
8. Honeydew melon
9. Kiwi
10. Cabbage
11. Watermelon
12. Mushrooms
13. Mangoes
14. Sweet potatoes
15. Carrots."

Nutrition advice can get very convoluted very fast, making it difficult for laypeople to sort out healthy foods from unhealthy ones. And it doesn't help clarify anything either that we are treated to the familiar non-stop cycle of "is coffee killing you?"/"is coffee saving your life?" type of contradictory and confusing media stories.

So, if there is a single rule of thumb I'd like to impart on the topic of nutrition, it's to ***avoid ultra-processed foods in general***—including the specific common ingredients in processed foods above—at all costs. They simply aren't worth the convenience and the taste factor when we consider what we know they do to long-term health.

Research published in the medical journal Nutrients [7] drew parallels between the rise in consumption of these food products—defined as "industrial formulations manufactured from substances derived from foods, which typically contain cosmetic and various other types of additive and little if any intact food"—in the Western developed world and increased rates of cancers, diabetes, and other chronic diseases:

> *"The prevalence of obesity and other diet-related chronic non-communicable diseases (NCDs), such as type II diabetes, hypertension, and some common cancers, is increasing*

> *worldwide. At the same time,* ***ultra-processed food production and consumption are steadily increasing in both high-income and lower-income countries****. Ultra-processed foods undermine food systems and dietary patterns based on minimally processed foods and freshly prepared meals.*
>
> ***Ultra-processed foods****, as defined by the NOVA food classification system, are not modified or merely processed foods... These products* ***are designed to be extremely palatable and convenient****, are often sold in large portion sizes, and are aggressively marketed.*
>
> *Analyses of nationally representative dietary surveys conducted in the United States, Canada, and Brazil consistently show that* ***high consumption of ultra-processed foods renders nutritionally unbalanced diets.****"*

Examples of ultra-processed foods many of us might have in our pantries or refrigerators and don't think twice about are canned soups, frozen dinners, soft drinks, candy, breakfast cereals, chicken nuggets, fast foods, and hot dogs.

Believe me when I tell you that I know firsthand and understand the pressures of modern life—the feeling of constantly being squeezed for time—and the convenience and ease that alluring ultra-processed foods offer. After all, they are engineered to appeal to our palates (sweet, salty, savory) and to require minimal prep on the consumer's part.

But, once again, we pay the price for that convenience and temporary pleasure with our long-term anti-aging health and eventually our lives.

For that reason, here are some basic dietary habits that I recommend instead, as an alternative to the standard American diet:

Balance your macronutrient ratios. The three macronutrients are carbohydrates, fats, and proteins. Your macronutrient ratio refers to the levels of intake of each of these relative to the others.

The exact right macronutrient for each will vary over time and from person to person depending on fitness goals, levels of physical activity, and individual genetics.

However, as a rule of thumb, carbohydrate intake should not exceed 50% of caloric intake—and, for weight loss, we should aim for a much lower percentage. Fat intake should account for about 30% of calories and protein around 20%.

Some people, including many of my patients, thrive on a ketogenic diet, a unique eating protocol that severely restricts carbohydrate intake to well below 50g per day.

Others do very well with a low-carbohydrate eating plan, which is typically defined as keeping carb intake to under 150 grams daily.

In any case, it's universally true that almost everyone who follows the standard American diet consumes far, far too many carbohydrates relative to healthy fats and protein, especially of the refined carbohydrate variety found in processed foods.

If and when you do consume carbohydrates in significant amounts, try to focus on complex carbs (a category which includes beans, whole grains, sweet potatoes, and fruits and veggies) rather than simple carbs (snacks and white breads, for example) because the former category of carbohydrate contains fiber that causes the carbs to digest more slowly, offer greater supplies of natural vitamins and minerals, and reduce blood sugar spikes.

- **Swap seed oils with healthier alternatives** like olive oil, avocado oil, coconut oil, or real butter (not margarine)
- **Eat the rainbow.** "Eat the rainbow" is an admittedly simplistic but nonetheless true maxim adopted by many nutritionists who focus on a natural diet. The wide spectrum of colors lent to various fruits and vegetables and other unprocessed foods are the result of the different phytonutrients (a term for nutrients sourced from plants) found in different foods.

So, get your blues via blueberries (an excellent low-carb fruit) and your reds from grapefruits and your greens from leafy veggies.

- **Eat as varied a diet as possible.** There are some foods that individuals may have an allergy to or intolerance to. In such cases, there may be medical interventions we can pursue to treat food intolerances, but for many patients it may very well be advisable to avoid them altogether.
  Beyond food intolerances, enjoying a wide range of foods not only ensures you're going to get a higher micronutrient intake, but it also helps support a more diverse, and therefore healthier, microbiome, by feeding a wider array of healthy bacteria—which, as we discussed before, it a critical and often overlooked component of overall health.
- **Place a premium on natural, whole foods.** Don't be fooled by tricky food labels: there is no standard for the designation or advertising of food products in the United States as "natural"; in fact, fully synthetic processed food products can and are legally labeled "natural" because there are enforcement mechanisms against deceptive marketing techniques.
  The best way to make sure that what you are eating is "natural" in the strict sense of the word is to eat, well, natural foods—fresh meats, veggies, and fruits, preferably sourced locally from a trusted farmer or rancher.

We've only just grazed the tip of the iceberg when it comes to adopting a healthier eating strategy, so this is by no means an exhaustive treatise of nutrition optimization. A compendium of current knowledge on optimal nutrition could fill volumes.

That said, optimizing your diet deserves much more consideration than a single chapter of my book.

If you are interested in further exploring how to turn food into medicine, pay me a visit. I always take the necessary time to discuss the importance of a healthy diet with my LowTE Florida patients, so don't be a stranger.

Wellness Factor #2: Prioritizing Slumber to Achieve Optimal Sleep

I get the pressures of daily living; I live in the modern developed world, too, after all. Sacrificing sleep when we all have a million things to do can often seem like the easiest thing to do to trim from the schedule and get everything done that we feel we need to.

But my expert advice is that skimping on sleep is a huge mistake for the reasons I'll explain now.

Shut-eye in sufficient quantity and quality is maximally important for long-term health and longevity. In fact, it's hard to exaggerate *how* important sleep is.

The U.S. Institute of Medicine Committee on Sleep Medicine and Research [] estimates that a shocking 70 million Americans—approximately one-fifth of the population—may, in fact, suffer from some form of sleep disorder:

> *"It is estimated that 50 to 70 million Americans chronically suffer from a disorder of sleep and wakefulness, hindering daily functioning and adversely affecting health and longevity. The cumulative long-term effects of sleep deprivation and sleep disorders have been associated with a wide range of deleterious health consequences including an increased risk of hypertension, diabetes, obesity, depression, heart attack, and stroke."*

We explored in the previous section the lamentably low, almost criminally low, amount of nutrition training that future doctors attending American medical schools receive, despite the central importance of diet to wellness and anti-aging.

Well, you may not be shocked to learn that the same phenomenon of inadequate training exists in the context of sleep in medical academia, as the Institute goes on to note:

> *"Although clinical activities and scientific opportunities in the field are expanding,* ***awareness among the general public and health***

> ***care professionals is low, given the magnitude of the burden***. *The available human resources and capacity are insufficient to further develop the science and to diagnose and treat individuals with sleep disorders. Therefore, the current situation necessitates a larger and more interdisciplinary workforce…*
>
> ***Renewed and revitalized commitments*** *to the field from the National Institutes of Health (NIH), academic health centers, private foundations, and professional societies* ***are essential to ensure appropriate public and professional awareness, education and training, basic and clinical research, and patient care***. *Finally, the fragmentation of research and clinical care currently present in most academic institutions requires the creation of accredited interdisciplinary sleep programs in academic institutions."*

Enter LowTE Florida—your premier interdisciplinary anti-aging health clinic! Here, we never overlook the importance of sleep.

Among the many impacts of poor sleep on health that may not seem obvious, not getting enough rest is a major drag on your metabolism—and may very well be one of the main reasons you struggle to lose weight.

Jessica Vogle, Certified Health Education Specialist, elaborates on the connection between metabolism and sleep through her work published at the National Wellness Institute [9]:

> *"Sleeping poorly, or not enough, slows the body's metabolism. Metabolism is the process by which the body converts calories to energy. Research suggests that* ***poor sleep makes the body's metabolism work less effectively, leaving more unexpended energy to be stored in the body as*** *fat.*
>
> ***Poor and insufficient sleep makes the body inclined to store calories as fat***. *Research indicates that poor sleep can trigger the body to make more insulin and cortisol. Higher insulin and cortisol*

levels appear to prompt the body to store energy as fat, especially in the abdomen.

***Poor sleep increases appetite**. **Not getting enough sleep**, and sleeping poorly, **leads to changes in hormones** that regulate hunger and feelings of fullness."*

So, when we're putting so much time and effort into getting your hormones in the correct balance via BHRT and supplementation, we'd be remiss not to prioritize sleep.

From a lifestyle standpoint, here are a few tactics you can use to improve sleep quality:

- Nix all caffeine-containing foods and drinks (coffee, tea, etc.) within six hours of bedtime. In addition to caffeine, the theobromine found naturally in chocolate can also act as a powerful stimulant and disrupt sleep, so it is best to avoid that as well. Also, nicotine right before bed is a no-no (and anyway you should quit smoking if you do for a whole host of other reasons as well!).
- Don't eat any carb-heavy meals within a few hours of bed. If possible, avoid eating at all after around 7 p.m.
- Turn off the phone/laptop/TV at least an hour before bed, as the blue lights and flicker rates on these devices can seriously disrupt your body's sleep-wake cycle. Read a book instead.
- Establish a consistent bedtime routine that includes, if possible, relaxation techniques of the kind we'll explore in the upcoming section.

But these are by no means all the ways that you can ensure optimal sleep, just the basics.

In addition to the patented LowTE Florida Sleep Deep supplement that I recommend to all my patients interested in improving their sleep duration and quality, bioidentical hormone replacement therapy using both bioidentical estrogen and testosterone is demonstrated to improve sleep quality in patients with hormone imbalances.

We have already referenced in this book the landmark study from the American Journal of Obstetrics and Gynecology [10], which found that "estrogen replacement therapy improved sleep quality, facilitated falling asleep, and decreased nocturnal restlessness and awakenings" and that "the more the subjects experienced insomnia, the better the estrogen replacement therapy facilitated falling asleep."

Bioidentical testosterone, for both men and women with deficiencies, is likewise proven to improve sleep quality.

Research published in the Journal of Clinical Endocrinology and Metabolism [11], which followed 1,300 men for three and a half years to measure the relationship between testosterone levels and sleep, found conclusive results pointing to the therapeutic application of bioidentical testosterone to improve sleep quality:

> *"Low total testosterone levels are associated with less healthy sleep in older men...*
>
> ***Lower testosterone levels... were associated with less consolidated sleep as demonstrated by decreased sleep efficiency and increased nocturnal awakenings**. Lower testosterone levels were **also associated with more severe sleep-disordered breathing**, as evidenced by a higher [apnea-hypopnea index] and more frequent hypoxemia*."*

*Hypoxemia is the clinical term for low oxygen saturation in the blood, which can be caused by sleep apnea, which in turn is tied to lower testosterone levels and a host of other negative health outcomes. We want to treat sleep apnea when it's identified—including potentially with bioidentical testosterone replacement therapy when appropriate—and we don't want chronic hypoxemia (defined as oxygen saturation below 95% for most people).

Using an all-of-the-above strategy relying on the aforementioned tools—supplementation, bioidentical hormone replacement therapy, and lifestyle changes—my patients benefit from reliable improvements in sleep.

Consider, for instance, LowTE Florida patient N.G.'s experience:

> *"I wanted to reach out to share my appreciation with Carolyn and your office. I have suffered with intense PMDD for the past three years, nothing I tried helped me.* ***It has been a month since I received my first dose of pellets****. My energy is amazing,* ***I am sleeping better... It's absolutely unbelievable the transformation in how I feel****. Thank you so much!"*
>
> -Nicole G.

Wellness Factor #3: Neutralizing Chronic Stress

Dovetailing nicely with the last section on sleep, as these issues are intertwined, minimizing chronic stress is also critical.

Chronic stress was already an epidemic in the West for many decades before 2020, but COVID-19 supercharged this ongoing public health disaster to previously unseen levels. You may have experienced this phenomenon yourself, which is presented in empirical data by a report from the American Psychological Association [12]:

> *"Despite several months of acclimating to a new reality and societal upheaval spurred by the COVID-19 pandemic, Americans are struggling to cope with the disruptions it has caused. Nearly 8 in 10 adults (78%) say the coronavirus pandemic is a significant source of stress in their life. And, 2 in 3 adults (67%) say they have experienced increased stress over the course of the pandemic.*
>
> *When considering the physical and emotional toll of increased stress, nearly* ***half of adults (49%) report their behavior has been negatively affected. Most commonly, they report increased tension in their bodies (21%), "snapping" or getting angry very quickly (20%), unexpected mood swings (20%), or screaming or yelling at a loved one (17%)."***

The pandemic era was, again, a noteworthy inflection point, but the trend of increasing chronic stress has been going on for many decades in America and will continue once COVID-19 is far in the rearview mirror. We see that reality reflected in statistics over time: the increasing rates of antidepressants and anti-anxiety drugs prescribed to tens of millions of Americans, rising suicide rates, etc.

All that to say: *Houston, we have a problem.*

But stress—what it is exactly and how it affects human health—is complicated and misunderstood.

So, before we get into how to effectively mitigate stress in your own life, let's unpack a few common misconceptions about what stress is and how harmful it is or isn't depending on the context.

Several forms of acute (meaning short-lasting) stress can actually be beneficial by stimulating your body to become stronger, more resilient, and/or more enthusiastic about life. These positive stressors (unless you overdo them, at which point they do more harm than good) potentially include:

- Exercise
- Cold exposure
- Heat exposure (more on that coming up)
- "The butterflies" you get before a first date or a big performance

These forms of positive acute stress can be powerful tools that temporarily (acutely) stimulate your nervous system and help you function at your best in moments of peak necessity.

The operative words here, though, are "positive" and "acute."

What we don't want is *chronic, negative* stress beyond our ability to manage and turn to our advantage, which not only robs us of joy in life but is also a killer on a long enough timeline.

The dysregulation of the neuroendocrine system—the nexus of the hormone system and the brain—is a key outcome of chronic unchecked stress.

Let's elaborate via clinical literature in Future Science OA [13]:

> *"Protracted, **stress-dependent neuroendocrine dysregulation may damage** directly or through functional circuits **practically all organs and tissues....***
>
> ***Diseases whose development has been linked to both stress and inflammation include cardiovascular dysfunctions, diabetes, cancer, autoimmune syndromes and mental illnesses** such as depression and anxiety disorders.*
>
> *Persistent, abnormal levels of cytokines and stress chemical mediators in the brain may also damage the parenchyma and cause neuronal death, thus contributing to the brain structural changes associated with chronic stress."*

I don't need to tell you all of this is bad news for those among us who struggle with chronic stress (which is many of us).

But it gets worse; stress itself isn't just detrimental to longevity and vitality, but it also drives epigenetic changes—epigenetics, being, as we have discussed before, changes to the expression of human DNA that can either promote health or cause disease.

Let's turn here to research published in Nature Reviews Genetics [14]:

> *"Accumulating **evidence points to a major role for chronic stress** of cell renewal systems **in the pathogenesis of** important human diseases, including **cancer, atherosclerosis and diabetes.** Here we discuss **emerging evidence that epigenetic abnormalities may make substantial contributions to these stress-induced pathologies.** Although the mechanisms remain to be fully elucidated, we suggest that **chronic stress can elicit heritable changes in the chromatin landscape that 'lock' cells in abnormal states, which then lead to disease...***

> *Both acute and **chronic stress can induce genetic and epigenetic changes** although, mathematically, they are more likely to occur during chronic stress.*
>
> *Thus, **adaptive pressure due to chronic stress could lead to the evolution of abnormal cell states that contribute to disease.**"*

It goes without saying, with all that clinical evidence established, that we surely need to treat chronic stress if that's an issue—and, as we've seen, it is a major issue for millions and millions of Americans.

For my patients with hormone imbalances, I've seen firsthand that simply getting the hormones taken care of through bioidentical hormone replacement therapy (BHRT) can do wonders for mitigating stress—which isn't surprising as hormone deficiencies are tied to excessive, chronic stress.

In addition to BHRT, many of our LowTE Florida patented supplements—like Citru-Slim with stress hormone-killing *Eurycoma Longifolia*—are also powerful stress-reduction tools.

Lifestyle practices, as well, can check stress of the mind and body, including:

- Eating healthy food and getting plenty of sleep (see prior sections of this chapter)
- Meditation
- Yoga
- Developing a strong spiritual foundation
- Breathing exercises
- Developing a plan for time management
- Therapy with a professional practitioner
- Cold exposure (i.e., cold showers, ice baths) *
- Heat exposure (sauna)*
- Learning how to say "no" and stick to it

*Acute, intentional cold and heat exposure produce, respectively, cold (CSPs) and heat shock proteins (HSPs), which are released in response to exposure to heat or cold and are increasingly understood to exert powerful neuroprotective effects, including protecting from the ravages of chronic stress, as explained by the Madame Curie Bioscience Database [15]:

> *"In response to many metabolic disturbances and injuries including stroke, neurodegenerative disease, epilepsy and trauma, the cell mounts a stress response with induction of a variety of proteins, most notably the 70 kD heat shock protein (Hsp70). The possibility that stress proteins might be neuroprotective was suspected because* ***Hsp70, in particular, was induced to high levels in brain regions that were relatively resistant to injury.*** *Hsp70 expression was also correlated with the phenomenon of induced tolerance. With the availability of transgenic animals and gene transfer, it has become increasingly clear that such* ***heat shock proteins do indeed protect cells from injury****. Several reports have now shown that selective overexpression of* ***Hsp70 leads to protection in several different models of nervous system injury****...*
>
> ***Hsp's chaperone functions may play a role in protection from injury*** *through improving the function of several different proteins. For instance, there may be a relationship between stress protein protection and oxidative injury...*
>
> *Recent studies in non-neuronal cell lines have shown that* ***Hsp70's protective effect may also be due to anti-apoptotic mechanisms****. Apoptosis, or programmed cell death is known to occur in pathological states either by activation of specific death receptors (Reviewed by Ashkenazi & Dixit72), or internally, via mitochondrial release of cytochrome c (Reviewed by Green & Reed73) ... Several papers have now established that* ***Hsps can interfere with apoptosis in various systems****...*
>
> *Recent studies from different laboratories have now established that the stress response provides the organism with a cellular*

process for self-preservation, and that ***stress proteins themselves can directly protect cells from death****. The specific mechanisms underlying this protection are not well understood, but are likely multifactorial, encompassing a wide range of cellular chaperone functions from the prevention of protein aggregation to interfering with various death cascades.* ***Capitalizing on the cell's natural response to stress is an attractive therapeutic target for a variety of nervous system diseases.****"*

The most common therapeutic method of heat exposure is sauna, while the most accessible method of cold exposure is cold showers or ice baths. I recommend both to my patients who are interested in improving their body's resilience to stress—but with important safeguards in place to avoid injury.

Beyond heat and cold exposure, each of the other above stress mitigation techniques on the list above deserves at least an entire chapter, if not a book, of its own, but we'll leave these there now for the sake of brevity.

I have recently started using an Infrared Sauna five days a week (twenty minutes at 150 degrees) and I notice (besides a huge sweat!) less stress, less body ache, improved mood, more compliments on my skin and looking youthful! I love my sauna! The research is crazy good on the benefits of regular sauna use.

As a holistic healthcare provider, I am always open to discussing these and the wide universe of other stress-reduction strategies with my LowTE Florida patients. There isn't, of course, a one-size-fits-all strategy that works for everyone, so it is likely your ideal stress management regimen would include some combination of the above.

Wellness Factor #4: Eliminating Exposure to Toxic, Hormone-Disrupting Chemicals

One question that many hormone replacement providers don't often ask but definitely should, which I do of my LowTE Florida patients, is: what lies at the root of hormone dysfunction in the first place, and how do we address those issues so that BHRT works as it's supposed to?

There are many environmental and genetic factors that combine to contribute to hormone imbalance, many of which we've already covered in this book. But a major factor that deserves special mention is the deluge of endocrine-disrupting chemicals (EDCs) in our everyday lives:

From the International Journal of Molecular Sciences [16]

> *"**Endocrine-disrupting chemicals (EDCs)** have significant impacts on biological systems, and **have been shown to interfere with physiological systems, especially by disrupting the hormone balance.** During the last few decades, EDCs have been shown to affect reproductive, neurological, and metabolic development and function and even stimulate tumor growth. EDC exposure during development can disrupt normal development patterns and alter susceptibility to disease. Many chemicals have endocrine-disrupting properties, including bisphenol A, organochlorines, polybrominated flame retardants, alkylphenols, and phthalates. **These compounds have gradually been elucidated as risk factors for many diseases, such as reproductive, neural, and metabolic diseases and cancers.**"*

It's no hyperbole to say that EDCs are literally *everywhere* in our environment, often in places that might not be immediately obvious, as explained by the National Institute of Environmental Health Sciences (NIEHS) [17]:

"Hormones act in extremely small amounts, and minor disruptions in those levels may cause significant developmental and biological effects...

Endocrine disruptors are found in many everyday products, including some cosmetics, food and beverage packaging, toys, carpet, and pesticides*. Some chemicals that act as flame retardants may also be endocrine disruptors.* ***Contact with these chemicals may occur through air, diet, skin, and water****. EDCs cannot be completely avoided or removed; however, you can make informed choices to reduce exposure and risk of any potential health effects."*

As noted above, as in the case of pesticide residue on foods, it's impossible to totally avoid EDCs, even in the most remote natural settings, as scientists now routinely discover contamination in the wild, far from any human population center. There is no hiding from EDCs; the only lasting solution will be achieved when he figures out how to remove these harmful chemical compounds from our environment.

However, in the meantime, here are a few basic steps you can take to reduce your and your family's exposure to EDCs:

- Purify your water using a high-quality filter
- Avoid plastic containers for food or drink whenever possible
- Opt for natural fabrics like cotton over synthetic ones like polyester or nylon
- Minimize your handling of receipts, which are commonly printed on paper with huge amounts of bisphenol-A, one of the most common EDCs
- Spring for fresh fruits and veggies over canned products whenever possible (and support your local farmers in the process!)
- Toss out your chemical-laden non-stick pots and pans in favor of stainless steel or cast-iron

Wellness Factor #5: Capitalizing on the Placebo Effect

In the context of stress and other stimuli, we have seen without a doubt that your psychological disposition and outlook (your thoughts and emotions) can have a negative effect on your health.

But, if negative thoughts and emotions can contribute to disease, which they can, why would it not logically follow that positive thoughts and emotions can contribute to health and wellness?

The so-called "placebo effect" in everyday life is real and potentially powerful when you harness it to your advantage.

In fact, the reason that clinicians include controlling factors for the placebo effect as a standard part of research studies is because it is *so* potent that it would throw off the results of experiments if not properly accounted for.

Let me explain.

We have referenced in this book many times by now the placebo effect, but here for the first time is a basic breakdown of the concept. More often than not, when conducting clinical trials of the kind that we have cited here in spades, researchers will separate the participants into two groups:

- The "experimental" group (the one receiving the real treatment under question)
- The "control" group (the one receiving a fake treatment, AKA placebo, often in the form of a sugar pill or a saline injection, that does not actually have any physiological activity in the body)

Once this model was instituted as standard practice in clinical work, researchers discovered quite a phenomenon: often, the placebo group experienced the same or even greater intended benefits of the treatment than the group that received the real thing!

So, what gives?

What's happening with the placebo effect is that the mind, which believes it is receiving real medicine even though what it's getting is just a sugar pill, convinces itself that the body is experiencing the physical benefits of a real drug or treatment, followed by either real or perceived health improvements.

It all boils down to perception: if we *really* believe, truly believe, that we are on the path to healing, our consciousness literally can't tell the difference between the real drug and the placebo because it's all the same.

A huge proportion of our health comes down to the power of the mind. Here's an iron law of the universe that you might not hear from your general medicine practitioner, because unfortunately (like nutrition) they don't teach much about the mind-body connection in medical school: getting yourself into the right frame of mind through intentional tweaking of your consciousness is absolutely indispensable for achieving peak mental and physical health.

Yes, the placebo effect is entirely a product of the human mind—but that doesn't make it any less real.

As meditation instructor Dr. Joe Dispenza often says, *you are the placebo*. Here is an apropos excerpt from his book by that name:

> *"Most change starts with the simple process of something outside of us altering something inside of us.* ***If you begin the inward journey and start to change your inner world of thoughts and feelings,*** *it should create an improved state of well-being. If you keep repeating the process in meditation, then in time, epigenetic changes should begin to alter your outer presentation—and* ***you become your own placebo.*** *"*

Of course, there's always going to be a role for medicine to play in improving health; if I didn't believe that I wouldn't be in clinical practice. But let's not pretend that the true path to wellness doesn't begin in the mind, with the unshakeable intention to improve your health and defy the aging process.

References

[1] Harvard T.H. Chan School of Public Health. (2017). Doctors need more nutrition education. Harvard T.H. Chan School of Public Health. https://www.hsph.harvard.edu/news/hsph-in-the-news/doctors-nutrition-education/

[2] Wartella E,, Lichtenstein, A., et al. (2010). Front-of-Package Nutrition Rating Systems and Symbols: Phase I Report. U.S. Institute of Medicine. https://www.ncbi.nlm.nih.gov/books/NBK209844/

[3] Totsch, S., Quinn, T., et al. (2017). The impact of the Standard American Diet in rats: Effects on behavior, physiology and recovery from inflammatory injury. Scandinavian Journal of Pain. https://pubmed.ncbi.nlm.nih.gov/28927908/

[4] Mai, B. and Liang-Jun, Y. (2019). The negative and detrimental effects of high fructose on the liver, with special reference to metabolic disorders. Diabetes, Metabolic Syndrome and Obesity. https://www.ncbi.nlm.nih.gov/pmc/articles/PMC6549781/

[5] Cleveland Clinic. (2020). Margarine or Butter: The Heart-Healthiest Spreads. https://health.clevelandclinic.org/margarine-or-butter-the-heart-healthiest-spreads-infographic

[6] EWG Science Team. (2024). EWG's 2024 Shopper's Guide to Pesticides in Produce™. https://www.ewg.org/foodnews/summary.php

[7] Rauber, F., da Costa Louzada, M., et al. (2018). Ultra-Processed Food Consumption and Chronic Non-Communicable Diseases-Related Dietary Nutrient Profile in the UK (2008–2014). Nutrients. https://www.ncbi.nlm.nih.gov/pmc/articles/PMC5986467/

[8] Colten, H. and Altevogt, B. (2006). Sleep Disorders and Sleep Deprivation: An Unmet Public Health Problem. Institute of Medicine (US) Committee on Sleep Medicine and Research. https://pubmed.ncbi.nlm.nih.gov/20669438/

[9] Vogle, J. (2023). Sleep Hygiene: Improve the Quality and Quantity of Sleep and Its Impact on Your Overall Well-Being. National Wellness Institute. https://nwijournal.com/sleep-hygiene-improve-the-quality-and-quantity-of-sleep-and-its-impact-on-your-overall-well-being/

[10] Polo-Kantola, P., Errkola, R. (1998). When does estrogen replacement therapy improve sleep quality? American Journal of Obstetrics and Gynecology. https://pubmed.ncbi.nlm.nih.gov/9609575

[11] Barrett-Connor, E., Dam, T., et al. (2008). The Association of Testosterone Levels with Overall Sleep Quality, Sleep Architecture, and Sleep-Disordered Breathing. The Journal of Clinical Endocrinology and Metabolism. https://www.ncbi.nlm.nih.gov/pmc/articles/PMC2453053/

[12] American Psychological Association. (2020). Stress in America™ 2020. American Psychological Association. https://www.apa.org/news/press/releases/stress/2020/report-october

[13] Mariotti, A. (2015). The effects of chronic stress on health: new insights into the molecular mechanisms of brain–body communication. Future Science OA. https://www.ncbi.nlm.nih.gov/pmc/articles/PMC5137920/

[14] Johnstone, S. and Baylin, F. (2010). Stress and the epigenetic landscape: a link to the pathobiology of human diseases? Nature Reviews Genetics. https://www.ncbi.nlm.nih.gov/pmc/articles/PMC3148009/

[15] Yenari, M. (2013). Heat Shock Proteins and Neuroprotection. Madame Curie Bioscience Database. https://www.ncbi.nlm.nih.gov/books/NBK6614/

[16] Changhwan, A., Eui-Bae, J. (2023). Endocrine-disrupting chemicals and disease endpoints. International journal of molecular sciences. https://pubmed.ncbi.nlm.nih.gov/36982431

[17] National Institute of Environmental Health Sciences (NIEHS). (n.d.). Endocrine Disruptors. National Institute of Environmental Health Sciences (NIEHS). https://www.niehs.nih.gov/health/topics/agents/endocrine

[18] Dispenza, J. (2014). You Are the Placebo: Making Your Mind Matter. Hay House, Inc.

Chapter XII

The Future of Anti-Aging Healthcare Is Full of Promise

I've done my best here to cover the waterfront of the state of anti-aging healthcare, reporting faithfully what I've learned and continue to learn regarding the latest research and exploring the most cutting-edge tools of the trade available to anti-aging practitioner like me—including but by no means limited to bioidentical hormone replacement therapy, strategic supplementation, cleaning up the diet, incorporating healthy lifestyle practices, and more.

So, where do we go from here?

If you're reading this in 2025 or beyond, take heart: you are living in a golden age of biomedical research, in which the rate of our understanding of anti-aging exponentially multiples with each passing year. AI, for whatever challenges it poses (a story for another book!), will undoubtedly accelerate our understanding of human aging and how to slow/prevent it even further.

Given how far we've come so far and where we're projected to go in the future, there is an ongoing scientific debate about whether aging can be accurately defined as a disease that can be cured, or even ultimately delayed indefinitely. Let's drop in a lengthy examination of this subject published in Trends in Molecular Medicine [1]:

> *"People over the age of 70 have multiple chronic diseases; for instance, based on autopsy records, the prevalence of prostate tumors in old men is nearly universal. Moreover, metabolic, immune, and cardiovascular dysfunctions, among others, affect the vast majority of elderly individuals. Even if no diseases are formally diagnosed, older individuals will often develop pre-*

clinical signs of these disorders. One can say that aging and disease go hand in hand: aging is a key risk factor for human chronic diseases, many treatments and interventions targeting age-related diseases can increase the lifespan of model organisms, and interventions extending organismal lifespan often delay diseases of aging. ***Is then aging a disease?***

The debate on the relationship between aging and disease is as old as our civilization, with many excellent researchers, philosophers, and practitioners supporting either side…

One criterion to decide whether aging is a disease is to determine if it, as a condition, is indeed treatable. The core issue here is to weigh-in viewing disease as a condition that affects a subset of the population (and can thus be 'treated') with the fact that aging affects everybody, and there is no evidence (at least in human populations) that it can be avoided. ***In medicine, whether a condition is a disease is often determined by how abnormal it is (e.g. how many standard deviations is it from the population norm?), and whether it leads to a decrement in quality of life****."*

On the first score, aging is certainly not abnormal, as it happens to us all at different rates and with different effects. But, on the second count, it certainly can and often does reduce the quality of life. So, it very well may be that we ought to consider aging a disease.

Ultimately, though, I'm not here to weigh in on such a weighty philosophical matter as whether aging should be classified as a disease or whether it's a natural process that we should accept as an integral part of the life-death cycle. That's a question for everyone to sort out on their own, in their own way, informed by their personal spiritual beliefs or lack thereof.

What I am here to tell you is that many of the ailments associated with aging that detract from quality of life and ultimately cause death are preventable—and many are curable. We can dramatically slow down, if not stop, the aging process to maximize vitality and longevity with an integrated anti-aging strategy, developed to meet the individual's needs based on personal genetics, health goals, etc.

That's what I do for my patients at LowTE Florida, and that's what we can do together when you make the call to embark on this journey with me. My door is always open.

References

[1] Gladyshev, T. and Gladyshev, V. (2016). A Disease or not a Disease? Aging as a Pathology. Trends in Molecular Medicine. https://www.ncbi.nlm.nih.gov/pmc/articles/PMC5540438/

Epilogue
Let's Get Started on Your Journey to Youthful Vitality Today

So, what does it take to get started living your best life?

Go to LowTEFlorida.com, complete the patient packet under BHRT and we will reach out to you to set up laboratory testing. Once we have the completed packet and your labs, we will then schedule your free telephone consultation with me. We will review your medical history, your symptoms you would like to correct, review your comprehensive labs line by line and we will map out a plan to get you feeling and looking your best! It is that simple...

I hope to see you soon at LowTE Florida!

~CZ